Experimental acute pancreatitis:
Models for testing a free radical mechanism

Peter Kruse

Ph.D.-thesis

Surgical Gastroenterologic Department D,
Copenhagen University Hospital Glostrup, and
Department of Pharmacology, University of Copenhagen
Denmark

Copenhagen, April 1997

Acknowledgements

This study was made from 1994 - 1997   during my employment as a research fellow at the Surgical Gastroenterologic Department, Copenhagen University Hospital, Glostrup and the Department of Pharmacology, the Panum Institute, University of Copenhagen. I sincerely wish to thank my supervisors Steen Boesby, Helge Worning and Henrik E. Poulsen for their constant support, invaluable to me during these years of research. I want to convey my special thanks to Henrik and to Steffen Loft for giving me access to excellent experimental facilities.

I learnt the basic skills in experimental surgery from two study tours: At the Department of Surgery, University of Lund, Sweden I visited Professor Ingemar Ihse and joined his fine experimental team led by Roland Andersson and Xiang-dong Wang. In Japan I visited two surgical departments led by Professor Yuji Nimura the First Department of Surgery, Nagoya University School of Medicine, Nagoya and Professor Masayuki Imamura the First Department of Surgery, Faculty of Medicine, Kyoto University. These visits enabled me to set up the animal models used in this study on my own.

I would like to thank the many people from the Department of Pharmacology, University of Copenhagen, for their help and advice. Special thanks to guest professor Mary Andersson, Sven Edelfors, Jens Lykkesfeldt and Anders Fuglsang for their help with my experiments. I am very grateful to the technicians who safely guided me through the laboratory jungle: Anna Hansen, Anni Jensen, Anette Hauman and Lise Reiff.   I wish to record my thanks to Ole Madsen and Steen Pedersen for their kind technical assistance. My   student colleagues Kirsten Vistisen, Helene Priemé, James Tuo and Michael Thomsen gave me pleasant companionship and lively discussions.

My sincere thanks also go to: Esther Hage and Dorte Hansen who made the histological scoring possible; Hans-Jørgen Skovgaard Jensen and Axel Kornerup Hansen who advised me on experimental techniques, animal welfare and ethics; Lars Horwarth and Michael Horwarth who build an infusion pump; my statistical teacher and counsellor Lene Theil Skovgaard who help me in avoiding statistical pitfalls; Kirsten Scharling and Gerda Holck for excellent literature searches; Lotte Clevin for medical illustrations and Sian Carstensen for language improvement.

This project would not have been possible without generous support from: The Danish Research Academy, Novo Nordisk Foundation, King Christian X's Foundation, Danish Foundation for the Advancement of Medical Science, Jacob Madsen and Olga Madsen's Foundation, Vibeke Binder and Povl Riis's Foundation, The Foundation of 1870, Reinholdt W. Jorck's Foundation and Jacob Johansen and   Maren Sophie Johansen's Foundation.

Last but not least, I wish to thank my lovely wife Flavia and my lively daughter Irene for putting up with their sometimes stressed and hard working husband and father.

Introduction

Acute pancreatitis in Denmark is a rather common disease and the incidence has increased in the period 1979 - 92 from 27 to 35/100.000/year in 1992 [1]. About 5 % of the patients develop severe necrotizing pancreatitis, and the overall lethality of patients with pancreatitis is 3.2 % [1]. The same tendency, but with slightly higher incidence, have been reported from Scotland [2] and Finland [3].

Technological development, especially in diagnostic imaging such as dynamic computed tomography and ultrasonography, has led to improved diagnostics of patients with acute pancreatitis. Although acute pancreatitis has been intensively researched, it is still a disease with an unclear pathogenesis and a lack of efficient treatment. Exactly 100 years ago, Chiari suggested that the digestive effect of the pancreatic juice could cause an intra-vital autodigestion of the pancreatic gland, thus being a possible reason to pancreatitis [4]. A relationship between acute pancreatitis and cholelithiasis was suggested by Opie in 1901 [5], and the influence of alcohol as a pathogenic factor by Symmers in 1917 [6]. The main causes of the disease are still considered to be cholelithiasis and alcohol. In three extensive papers in 1889, Fitz [7] described and characterised the disease, and his description looks as if it was taken from a modern textbook of surgery.

Today, when patients develop acute pancreatitis, especially in the severe form, only intensive supportive treatment and surgical intervention is available. Because the initial pathophysiological events are still unknown, specific pharmacological therapy is not yet available to these patients. Indeed, a great amount of research has been done to understand the cellular events during the disease in order to discover new treatment modalities [8]. To study early events of acute pancreatitis, several experimental models using animals have been developed, but only recently, have guidelines for standardisation of the different models been published [9].

Oxygen radicals have been suggested an important pathogenetic factor in many diseases such as arteriosclerosis, chronic inflammatory diseases, diseases involving ischemia/reperfusion, cataract and many more [10]. In gastrointestinal disorders such as intestinal ischemia, inflammatory bowel disease, gastric ulcer, pancreatitis and others, an involvement of oxygen radicals has been proposed [11].

Since Sanfey in 1984 [12] suggested a role of oxygen derived radicals in experimentally induced pancreatitis, many attempts have been made to clarify their importance. Indeed, such an involvement of oxygen radicals would be interesting, because a potential treatment with the use of antioxidants would be possible.

Background

Models of experimental acute pancreatitis

In the attempt to model the human disease, several experimental models of acute pancreatitis (AP) have been developed in a variety of animals [13]. The models can be divided into "direct" and "indirect" varieties according to whether the techniques require abdominal surgery and manipulation of the organs or not.

Most of the *direct models* are designed to mimic the clinical situation of gallstone induced AP. The "Duct infusion model" (DI) is one of the most often studied direct models in which retrograde injection of bile acids, (such as taurocholate) into the pancreatobiliary duct (PBD), creates a necrotizing AP [14]. The proposed contents of the infusion liquid are numerous: olive oil, conjugated and unconjugated bile acids, activated enzymes, detergents etc. Anterograde perfusion of the PBD is used in the "Pancreatic duct perfusion model" [15]. Another way of increasing the intraductal pressure is by ligating the PBD, as in the "Duct occlusion model" (DOC), leading to a less severe pancreatitis compared with the DI-model [16]. But the severity can be increased by combining this model with hyperstimulation of the pancreas, as mentioned below [17]. Surgical closure of the proximal and the distal part of duodenum is followed by reflux of duodenal content into the pancreas. This procedure gives rise to a necrotizing AP as in the "Closed duodenal loop model" (CDL) [18]. Some of the direct models have been designed to mimic AP due to ischemia/reperfusion (ISC) by clamping the pancreatic arteries or veins [19, 20] or by injecting microspheres into the vascular bed of the pancreas [21]. In the "Ex-vivo perfusion model" (EXP), the pancreas is isolated and the vascular system is cannulated together with the PBD and then AP can be induced in several ways (by ischemia, by hyperstimulation etc.) [22].

As *indirect models* the most studied one is the "Secretagogue model" (SEC), based on the effect of hyperstimulation of the pancreas by cholecystokinin (CCK) receptor agonists, such as CCK, cerulein or cholinesterase. The effect of hyperstimulation with cerulein is species dependent and in rats the result is an edematous AP [23]. By feeding a choline-deficient ethionine rich diet (CDE) to young female mice, a late and very severe necrotizing AP develops [24]. Feeding an ethionine-supplemented diet to other animals results only in an edematous AP [25]. Rarely used models are the "immunologic models" where animals are sensitised to an antigen followed by an additional antigen provocation leading to AP [26].

Reactive oxygen species

A free radical is defined by Halliwell and Guterridge, as " any species capable of independent existence that contains one or more unpaired electrons" [10]. During the normal oxygen metabolism 95 % of O_2 is transformed to water. The remaining 5 % of the oxygen undergoes only a step-wise one-electron reduction and becomes the major source of free radicals (Figure 1). As described by Halliwell [27], a superscript dot is used to denote free radicals.

Ground state oxygen, though not very reactive, is a biradical having two unpaired electrons. Additional input of energy can change the orbital position of these electrons, thus creating two forms of singlet oxygen, sigma and delta oxygen. Sigma singlet oxygen has two unpaired electrons and is therefore a radical, however, delta singlet oxygen has no unpaired electrons and is not a radical [10].

A one electron reduction of molecular oxygen generates the superoxide anion radical $O_2^{-\bullet}$. The further reduction by two electrons of molecular oxygen produces the peroxide ion (O_2^{2-}), which in the protonated form is hydrogen peroxide (H_2O_2). Hydrogen peroxide is not a free radical, nevertheless, it is harmful to cells since it can cross cell membranes and be a source of the most reactive molecule, the hydroxyl radical ($^\bullet OH$). The tri-electron reduction of molecular oxygen gives the hydroxyl radical which has a very short half life and thus a short radius of action (30 Å) [28]. The metal-catalysed Fenton reaction is a main source of $^\bullet OH$. In this reaction Fe^{3+} is reduced to Fe^{2+} that reacts with H_2O_2, thus producing $^\bullet OH$ [10]. Figure 1 shows the full four-electron reduction of oxygen to water and the step-wise one-electron reduction.

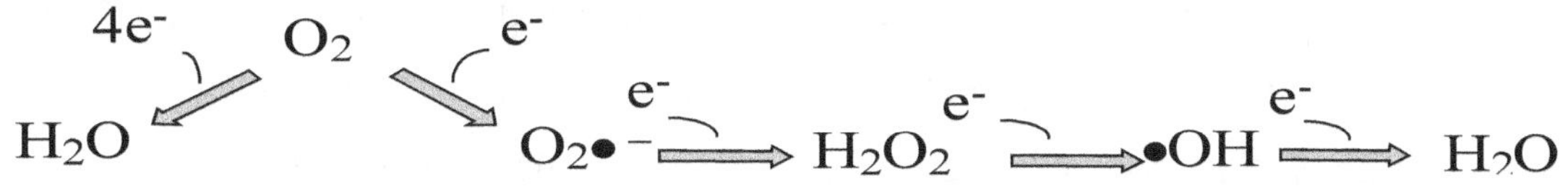

Figure 1. The four electron reduction of oxygen directly to H₂O (left) or step-wise as univalent reduction (right)

Since most of the biological relevant compounds with radical activity are derived from molecular oxygen, but not all have radical nature, such as H_2O_2 and delta singlet oxygen, a designation is often used: reactive oxygen species (ROS). In Table 1, different examples of ROS are listed together with their estimated half-lives.

Table 1. Reactive oxygen species (modified from [29])

Species	Common name	Half-life (37C)
$^\bullet OH$	Hydroxyl radical	1 nanosecond
$HO_2^\bullet$	Hydroperoxyl radical	unstable
$O_2^{-\bullet}$	Superoxide radical	enzymatic
$^1O_2$	Singlet oxygen	1 microsecond
$RO^\bullet$	Alkoxyl radical	1 microsecond
$ROO^\bullet$	Peroxyl radical	7 seconds
$NO^\bullet$	Nitric oxide	1-10 seconds
H_2O_2	Hydrogen peroxide	stable
$HOCl$	Hypochlorous acid	stable
$ONOO^-$	Peroxynitrite	2 seconds #
--		

R=lipid for example linoleate. A superscript dot (') is used to denote a free radical
From reference [30]

Defence systems against ROS

Because ROS are constantly being produced, organisms have an extensive protection system in the extra- and intracellular antioxidants. Antioxidants, or scavengers, are defined as " any substance that when present at low concentrations, compared with those of the oxidizable substrate, considerably delays or inhibits oxidation of the substrate" [31]. The antioxidants can be divided into enzymatic and non-enzymatic compounds and the latter can further be divided into exogenous (dietary) and endogenous (synthesised in the body). The major enzymatic antioxidants consist of superoxide dismutase (SOD), catalase (Cat) and glutathione peroxidase (Gpx). Table 2 shows some of the enzymatic antioxidants and the reactions they catalyze: SOD is found in mitochondria and cytosol and converts superoxide to hydrogen peroxide. Cat is found in peroxisomes in most tissue and serves to remove hydrogen peroxide.

Gpx is found in the cytosol of the cells and reduces hydrogen peroxide to water by oxidizing glutathione (GSH) into its oxidized form, glutathione disulfide (GSSG) [10].

Table 2. Major enzymatic antioxidants

Enzymes	Reaction
Superoxide dismutase (SOD)	$2\,O_2^{\bullet-} \;+\; 2\,H^+ \;\rightarrow\; H_2O_2 \;+ O_2$
Catalase (Cat)	$2\,H_2O_2 \;\rightarrow\; 2\,H_2O + O_2$
Glutathione peroxidase (Gpx)	$H_2O_2 + 2\,GSH \;\rightarrow\; GSSG + 2\,H_2O$

GSH = reduced glutathione, GSSG = oxidized glutathione

A selection of some of the non-enzymatic antioxidants in humans is shown in Table 3. Both the endogenous and exogenous antioxidants are able to neutralise free radicals, and also metal binding proteins are able to sequester iron and copper ions which if free, can catalyse oxidative reactions. The two most important non-enzymatic antioxidants are GSH and ascorbic acid (AA) [32, 33]. GSH, a water-soluble tripeptide, is mainly found in the cytosol and in the mitochondria [10]. As a major contributor to the reducing environment in tissue, GSH can scavenge hydrogenperoxide and other peroxides [34]. Besides the scavenging capacity of GSH, it is important in maintaining the intracellular redox state via the GSH/GSSG-ratio [35]. The redox state of pancreatic acinar cells is critical for proper protein folding in the endoplasmic reticulum [36, 37], the integrity of the cytoskeleton [38] and the acinar stimulus secretion-coupling [39, 40]. The concentration of GSH in a rat's pancreas is about 2 μmol/g wet weight, being less than in the liver, kidney and small intestine. Rat plasma values are around 20-30 μM [41]. The overall cellular ratio of GSSG/GSH in healthy rats is from 1 - 3 % [36]. GSH is closely related with the metabolism of AA and both substances can spare the other [42, 43].

AA, or vitamin C, is water soluble and is found in both the cytosol, plasma and other body fluids [44]. AA can scavenge oxygen-, nitrogen- and sulphur-centered radicals [45]. The concentration of AA in rat pancreas is about 10 - 20 nmol/mg protein, higher in the endocrine than in the exocrine part, and in plasma about 100 μM [46, 47]. In human plasma AA was found to be the most important antioxidant as AA = protein-thiols>bilirubin>urate>α-tocopherol [48, 49]. Only when AA was totally depleted in plasma, and other antioxidants were partially depleted, was a rise in lipid peroxidation seen [33]. Other important water soluble antioxidants are cysteine, uric acid and bilirubin and as lipid soluble antioxidants tocopherols and carotenoids [31]. α-tocopherol (Vitamin E) is an important lipid soluble antioxidant, that co-operatively interacts with ascorbic acid against oxidation of lipids [50].

Table 3. Components of non-enzymatic antioxidants in humans (modified from [29])

Endogenous antioxidants	Dietary antioxidants	Metal binding proteins
NADPH and NADH	Vitamin C (ascorbic acid)	Ceruloplasmin (copper)
Glutathione and thiols (-SH)	Vitamin E (tocopherols)	Metallothionein (copper)
Ubiquinol (coenzyme Q)	Carotenoids	Albumin (copper)
Uric acid	Flavonoides	Transferrin (iron)
Bilirubin	Polyphenols	Ferritin (iron)
Metalloenzymes	_ _	Myoglobin (iron)
_ _		_ _

When the level of ROS exceeds the capacity of the defence systems, oxidative stress occurs with possible damage to cellular components such as lipids, proteins and DNA [31]. The oxidative stress can be monitored by measuring the loss of antioxidants [31] or by measuring markers of lipid peroxidation [51] such as malondialdehyde (MDA) and conjugated dienes (CD), and markers of DNA-damage such as 8-oxo-7.8-dihydro-2'-deoxoguanosine (8-oxodG), i.e., a free radical induced modification of the DNA base guanine [52].

Sources of ROS in experimental acute pancreatitis

The pathogenesis of pancreatitis in different experimental models varies and is mostly still unclear. But in all models, an initial injury, whether toxic, due to ischemia/reperfusion or hyperstimulation, leads to an activation of the pancreatic digestive enzymes which results in various degrees of acinar cell damage, interstitial edema and inflammatory response [53, entire suppl.]. This injury can possibly promote the production of ROS through at least three mechanisms: Damage to the electron transferring chains (i.e., the mitochondrial respiratory chain or the microsomal electron transferring chain), activation of polymorphonuclear leukocytes (PMN's) or activation of the xanthine oxidase system, as a result of ischemia/re-perfusion.

The electron transport chains in the mitochondria and in the endoplasmic reticulum are considered to be one of the most important sources of superoxide radical in vivo in most aerobic cells [10] and their damage may lead to an increased formation of ROS [54]. Impairment of mitochondrial function is related to the severity of the pancreatic injury in some models such as the cerulein induced AP [56].

It has been suggested that ROS triggers the accumulation of PMN's to damaged tissue. This may lead to "leukocyte sticking" of the capillary walls and even plugging of the entire vessel lumina, thus resulting in impaired microcirculation [57]. Damage of the host tissue by the PMN's may occur through different mechanisms while they migrate to the damaged tissue. These include premature activation during migration, extracellular release of microbicidal products, removal of damaged host cells or failure to terminate the acute inflammatory response [57]. Activated PMN's have a 50- to 100-fold increased oxygen consumption, called the "respiratory burst", leading to the production of cytotoxic ROS [57]. In experimental AP in rats, however, PMN's appear to be involved in a rather late stage of the disease (> 9 hours) [58, 59]. Most of the experimental studies suggest an early damage by ROS in the development of experimental acute pancreatitis. Therefore, the "respiratory burst" from activated PMN's may not be an important initial mechanism to the production of ROS. Circulating activated PMN's have been found in other organs (for instance lungs [60, 61]) and could be an important factor for the associated multiple organ failure seen in AP [62, 63].

Ischemia/reperfusion depletes tissue adenosine triphosphate, ATP, and causes accumulation of hypoxanthine. This hypoxanthine is oxidized by xanthine oxidase thus generating ROS [10]. The reoxygenation injury caused by these ROS is seen in diseases like myocardial ischemia, during organ transplantation and after a stroke (cerebral ischemia) [64]. In experimental AP the role of ROS originating from ischemia/reperfusion seems to depend on the different experimental designs   [65]. In ex-vivo perfused canine pancreatitis   models, pre-treatment with allopurinol, a xanthine oxidase inhibitor, attenuates the injury process [66], whereas allopurinol given after the onset of the disease fails to change the progression of the injury   [67].

Evidence of ROS involvement in acute pancreatitis

Animal studies

In the majority of   animal studies, the preferred species have been rodents (mice and rats) with only a few studies performed on other species such as dogs. Since Sanfey proposed a possible involvement of ROS in experimental acute pancreatitis [12], the subject has mainly been investigated in three directions:

1) Direct measurement of ROS using electron spin resonance (ESR) or chemiluminescence has been used in only a few studies due to the great difficulties involved in these techniques; these studies are summarised in Table 4. Because free radicals have the property of paramagnetism, they can be detected even in very small concentrations by ESR. The only ESR study performed in regarding AP, has shown a rise in hydroxyl radical concentration after 12 hours in a CDE model in mice   [68]. Chemiluminescence shows free radical production, i.e., an increase in chemiluminescence, between 0.2 and 12 hours after induction of AP   [69-71].

Table 4. Direct measurements of ROS in experimental AP. Each study is presented with animals, models (outlined in page 6) and recorded variables. As major findings, ↑ indicates an increase in concentration and ↓ indicates a decrease.

Author	*Animal*	*Model*	*Measurements*	*Major findings*
Gough [69]	Rats	SEC:Cerulein	Chemiluminescence	↑ 20 min.
		DI:Taurochol.		↑ 15 min.
Kishimoto [70]	Rats	SEC:Cerulein	Chemiluminescence	↑ 2 -3 h
Murakami [63]	Rats	DI: Bile + trypsin	Chemiluminescence	↑ 2 -3 h in lungs
Nonaka [68]	Mice	CDE	ESR	OH-adduct ↑ 12 h
Peralta [71]	Rats	CDL	Chemiluminescence	↑ 6 -12 h

2) In interventional studies, specific scavengers, such as SOD and catalase, are used in order to "detoxify" ROS. Thereafter evaluate the effects on histology and/or activities of pancreatic enzymes are evaluated. In many of these studies, being the dominant part of the literature concerning this topic, the animals were pre-treated with scavengers before induction of AP. The effect of scavenger treatment varies from positive to none, depending on the type of the chosen experimental model. The overall result indicates a possible involvement of ROS in most of the mentioned experimental models as summarised in Table 5.

Table 5. Experimental AP and interventional studies. The table shows the animals, models (outlined in page 6) and scavenger used in each study. Alterations in histological variables, such as edema, parenchymal necrosis etc, and in lipase and/or amylase activities in plasma, are described according to the outcome: positive or none.

Author	Animal	Model	Scavenger	Histology	Enzymes
Sanfey [12, 66]	Dogs	EXP	SOD/catalase, allopurinol	Less edema	Positive
Nordback [72]	Dogs	EXP	SOD, Cat	Positive	Positive
Guice [73]	Rats	SEC:Cerulein	SOD/Cat	Positive	Not measured
Wisner [74]	Rats	SEC:Cerulein	PEG-SOD	Positive	Positive
Schoenberg [75]	Rats	SEC:Cerulein	SOD/Cat	Positive	None
Wisner [76]	Rats	SEC:Cerulein	Allopurinol	Less edema	Positive
Sledzinski [77]	Rats	SEC:Cerulein	4-OH-TEMPO	Positive	Not measured
Nonaka [78]	Mice	SEC:Cerulein	2-0-octadecyl-ascorbicacid	Positive	Positive
Steer [79]	Rats	SEC:Cerulein	SOD/PEG-SOD,Cat, allopurinol, DMSO	Less edema	None
	Mice	CDE		Less edema	None
Niederau [80]	Mice	SEC:Cerulein	SOD/Cat	Less edema	None
			Allopurinol	None	None
			DMSO	None	None
Schoenberg [81]	Rats	SEC:Cerulein	SOD/Cat	+ on necrosis	None
	Rats	DI:Taurochol.		- on inflam. and edema	Positive
Niederau [80]	Rats	DI:Taurochol.	SOD/Cat	None	Positive
			Allopurinol	None	None
			DMSO	None	None
Closa [82]	Rats	DI:Taurochol.	SOD, indometacine	No effect on edema	None
Wang XD [83]	Rats	DI:Taurochol.	NAC	Less edema	None
Blind [84]	Rats	DI:Taurochol.	SOD/Cat	Less edema	None
Lankisch [85]	Rats	DI:Taurochol.	Allopurinol	None	None
	Mice	CDE		None	None
Rutledge [86]	Mice	CDE	Cat, allopurinol, DMSO	None	None
Nonaka [87]	Mice	CDE	2-0-octadecyl-ascorbic acid	(Improved survival)	Positive
Niederau [80]	Mice	CDE	SOD/Cat	Less edema	Positive
			Allopurinol	None	None
			DMSO	None	None
Hirano [88]	Rats	DOC +ISC	Protease inhib., SOD	Positive	Positive
Koiwai [89]	Rats	DOC	SOD/Cat, allopurinol	Positive	Positive
Peralta J [71]	Rats	CDL	SOD	None on edema	None
Tsimoyiannis [90]	Rats	CDL	SOD, Cat, allopurinol, DMSO	Positive DMSO: no effect	Positive DMSO: no effect

3) Studies measuring endogenous scavengers during AP, such as the enzymatic scavengers SOD, Cat, Gpx and the non enzymatic scavenger GSH, are few. As markers of damage due to free radicals, lipid peroxidation products, such as MDA or conjugated dienes, have been measured. Cerulein, choline deficient ethionine rich diet and common duct occlusion induced AP in rodents seems to deplete scavengers such as SOD, Cat and GSH within 4 - 6 hours, while an increase of makers of lipid peroxidation occurred after 3 - 6 hours. A much faster model is the taurocholate induced AP in rats where changes are seen after 0.5 hours. Other important scavengers, such as ascorbic acid, and other markers of damage to cellular protein or DNA due to ROS, have not been investigated. The studies are summarised in Table 6.

Table 6. Experimental AP and measurements of scavengers in pancreatic tissue. Each study is presented with animals, models (outlined in page 6) and recorded variables. As major findings, ↑ indicates an increase in concentration and ↓ indicates a decrease.

Author	Animal	Model	Measurements	Major findings
Lüthen [91]	Rabbits	SEC:Cerulein + ethanol	GSH, GSSG	No changes compared to controls
Dabrowski [92]	Rats	SEC:Cerulein	MDA, SOD	MDA ↑ SOD ↓ after 3 h
Dabrowski [93]	Rats	SEC:Cerulein	MDA, -SH groups	MDA ↑ SH-groups ↓ after 6 h
Schoenberg [75]	Rats	SEC:Cerulein	MDA, CD	CD ↑, MDA ↑ after 3.5 h
Lüthen [94]	Rats	SEC:Cerulein	GSH, GSSG	GSH ↓ after 4 h GSSG no increase
Nonaka [95]	Mice	SEC:Cerulein	LPO, SOD, Cat, Gpx	LPO ↑ after 6 h SOD ↓ after 6 h Cat ↓ after 9 h Gpx ↑ after 9 h
Neuschwander-Tetri [96]	Mice	SEC:Cerulein	GSH	GSH ↓ after 4 h
Schoenberg [97]	Rats	DI:Taurochol.	MDA, GSH, GSSG	MDA ↑ after 0.5 h GSH ↓ after 0.5 h GSSG ↑ after 3.5 h
Dabrowski [98]	Rats	DI:Taurochol.	MDA, SH-groups, SOD, Cat	MDA ↑ after 1 h SH-groups ↓ after 1 h SOD ↓ after 1 h Cat ↑ after 1 h
Koiwai [89]	Rats	DOC	MDA	MDA ↑ after 6 h
Nonaka [99]	Mice	CDE	LPO, SOD	LPO ↑ after 6 h SOD ↓ after 8 h

Human studies

Clinical studies on the involvement of ROS in AP are scarce, and the researchers have only included a limited number of patients. Assessments of scavengers, such as GSH and AA, show lower levels in patients with AP compared with controls. Only in one study the authors described the changes in the pancreatic tissue in patients with AP [100]; MDA in pancreas was high with pancreatic GSH depleted but with no increase in GSSG. In patients with AP markers of lipid peroxidation in plasma, such as MDA, are increased compared with control patients. As a quantitative measure of ROS, chemiluminescence in whole blood from AP patients was increased compared with controls [101]. Altogether, these findings suggest an involvement of ROS in human AP, but they do not determine whether ROS is the cause or the result of AP in humans. Results from human studies are summarised in Table 7.

Table 7. Evidence of ROS involvement in human AP. Each study is presented with the number of patients and the recorded variables. As major findings, ↑ indicates an increase in concentration and ↓ indicates a decrease.

Author	Measurements	Major findings
Schoenberg [100] (n=9)	MDA, CD, GSH/GSSG	Tissue and plasma MDA ↑, tissue-GSH ↓, and tissue-GSSG and CD were unchanged in patients with AP versus controls
Braganza [102] (n=42)	AA, selenium, β-carotene, α-tocopherol and LPO	All antioxidants ↓ and LPO ↑ in patients with AP versus controls
Waele [103] (n=20)	AA, α-tocopherol	Plasma AA and plasma α-tocopherol ↓ in patients with AP versus controls
Scott [104] (n=29)	AA	Plasma AA ↓
Guyan [105] (n=10)	LPO, CD, fluorescence	All variables in plasma ↑ in patients with AP versus controls
Honjo [106] (n=6)	LPO, α-tocopherol, Gpx	Plasma LPO ↑, plasma α-tocopherol and plasma Gpx ↓ in patients with AP versus controls
Kuklinski [107] (n=8)	MDA	Plasma MDA ↑ in patients with AP versus controls
Schofield [108] (n=18)	GSH	Plasma GSH ↓ in patients with AP versus controls
Lu [101] (n=12)	Chemiluminescence of whole blood	Chem. ↑ in patients with AP versus controls

Overview

From both animal and human research on acute pancreatitis, summarised in Tables 4 - 7, some involvement of ROS is evident, but the importance of these reactive species is still unclear. Direct measurements of ROS in animals show an early involvement (within hours). If animals are treated with scavengers, the outcome of the induced AP seems to be improved in most but not in all the models. Measurements of cellular scavengers and of markers of oxidative damage in animals during AP also indicate an early involvement of ROS. But only a few studies have measured both reduced and oxidized antioxidants and at the same time markers of oxidative damage in the cells. Studies on human AP have also suggested an involvement of ROS. But due to difficulties in tissue sampling there is only weak evidence regarding the mechanisms and the site of the initial pathophysiological changes. Furthermore, data from human AP does not display the very early stages of the disease, as the patients are admitted to the hospital several hours after onset of the disease.

Thus, in order to investigate the involvement and the importance of ROS in the early events of AP, time course studies on different animal models, such as models resembling necrotizing and edematous AP in humans, remains to be conducted. Reduced and oxidized major antioxidants in both plasma and tissue compartments should be assessed along with relevant markers of oxidative damage to the cells, such as products of lipid peroxidation and DNA oxidation.

Hypothesis and aims

Based on the current literature, a free radical mechanism is suggested as an early event in acute experimental pancreatitis. We hypothesized that induction of acute pancreatitis would lead to:

- an early depletion of antioxidants
- a simultaneous rise in the oxidized antioxidants
- and a rise in a marker of lipid peroxidation and a marker of DNA oxidation

To enable us to test our hypothesis, we conducted this study in two parts:

In *Part I* we intended to:

- Characterize a direct model of acute pancreatitis (Taurocholate model) through a time course and a dose response study

- Characterize an indirect model of acute pancreatitis (Cerulein model) through a time course study

In *Part II* we intended to:

- Conduct an initial study, to evaluate scavenger levels, the relevant time course, sampling techniques and assays

- Conduct a study on the two pancreatitis models to measure the early changes in the levels of ascorbic acid, glutathione and their oxidized forms, and a marker of lipid peroxidation and DNA oxidation.

Part I: Characterization of two rat models

In the laboratory we wanted to characterize two rat models of AP; a direct model (the taurocholate duct infusion model) and an indirect model (the cerulein infusion model). We followed the recently published guidelines for standardization of experimental AP [109]. The taurocholate model was carried out with a time course and a dose-response study, while the cerulein model was carried out only with a time course study as sufficient dose-response studies are available from the literature [110].

Materials and methods

Animals: Adult male Wistar rats (Pan:WIST) were kept on aspen bedding (Tapvei), one to a cage (Makrololen, Type III), fed standard pelleted rat diet (Altromin 1314 ®, Denmark), and subjected to regular 12 hour light-dark cycles. The air was changed 12-14 times/hr, the room temperature was 21-23 °C and the relative humidity was 45 - 70 %.The rats were fasted for 12 hours before the operation, but had free access to water.

Anesthesia and analgesia: The animals were anaesthetized with halothane/N_2O/O_2 (1.5%-/50%/50%). At the end of each operation, repeatedly if necessary, the animals received buprenorphine subcutaneously (Anorfin ®, GEA, Copenhagen) 0.2 mg/kg body weight (BW) to relieve postoperative pain [111].

Induction of acute pancreatitis in taurocholate model (modified from [14, 112], Figure 2*)*: During anesthesia the rats were placed supinely on a heating pad (body temperature: 38.0 ± 0.5 °C). The abdomen was opened through a midline incision and the pancreatico biliary duct (PBD) was cannulated transduodenally (24 G Neoflon®, Ohmeda, Sweden). We placed a micro vascular clamp (20 g/mm² clamp pressure) on the duct at the hilum of the liver. A 6-0 nylon ligature was tightened around the cannula and the wall of the duct, close to the duodenum, to prevent back flow. We infused taurocholate diluted in isotonic saline with a volume of app. 250 µl (0.1 ml/100 g BW, taurocholic acid, sodium salt, Sigma T-0750), into the PBD, with an infusion pump (infusion speed: 0.1 ml/min, Braun Perfusor®, Germany, coefficient of variation of 2.1 %). The ligature, the cannula and finally the clamp were removed thus leaving the PBD intact. The duodenal perforation was closed with a 6-0 nylon purse string suture and the abdominal wall with a 4-0 nylon suture. In all the procedures, we focused on a-traumatic surgical techniques. In the dose-response study, we applied a minor modification to minimize manipulation of the pancreas: the ligature around the cannula was replaced by a microtube clamp (Modified Acland clamp, TC-1, S&T, Switzerland).

Induction of acute pancreatitis in cerulein model (modified from [113], *Figure 3)*: Cerulein was purchased from Sigma Chemicals, St. Louis, USA (Sigma no: C-9026).

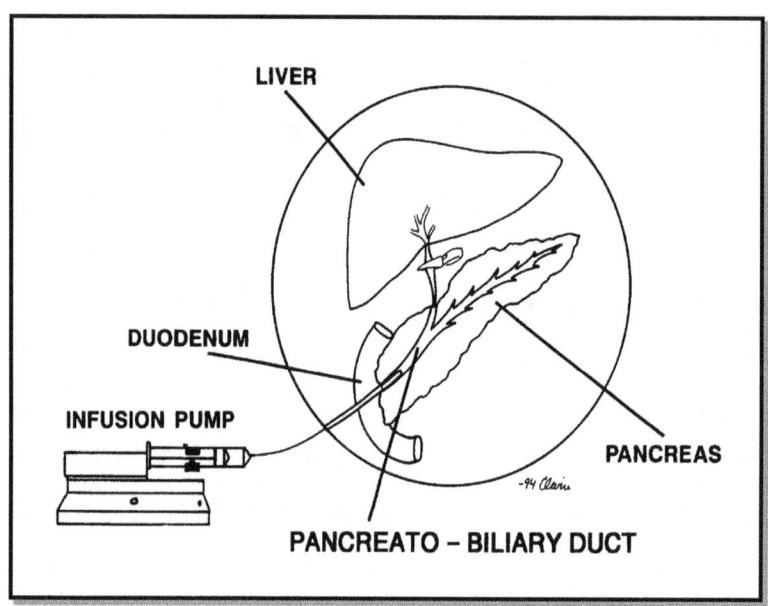

Figure 2. Taurocholate model

The compound was weighed and dissolved in physiological saline adjusted to pH 7.4 with ammonium hydroxide 0.01 M. We used 24 hour mini-osmotic pumps from Alzet ® (Model 2001D, mean pumping rate 9.2 ± SD 0.3 µl/hr, mean fill volume 221 ± SD 7 µl). Each pump was attached to a polyethylene tube with an inner diameter of 0.38 mm and an outer diameter of 0.76 mm (Tygon ®, Norton Plastics, Akron, USA) and was quality controlled by weighing to assure correct output. The pumps were filled using sterile techniques and presoaked in physiologic saline three hours before insertion.

After the induction of anesthesia, the rats were placed supinely on a heating pad (constant body temperature, 38.0 ± 0.5 °C) and incised over the external jugular vein and on the back. We placed a prefilled and presoaked pump subcutaneously in the mid scapular region and tunneled the catheter subcutaneously to the jugular vein. We inserted the catheter 2 cm into the vein with the tip placed just above the heart and ligated the proximal and distal part of the vein with 4-0 silk. We closed the skin incisions with nylon 4-0 suture.

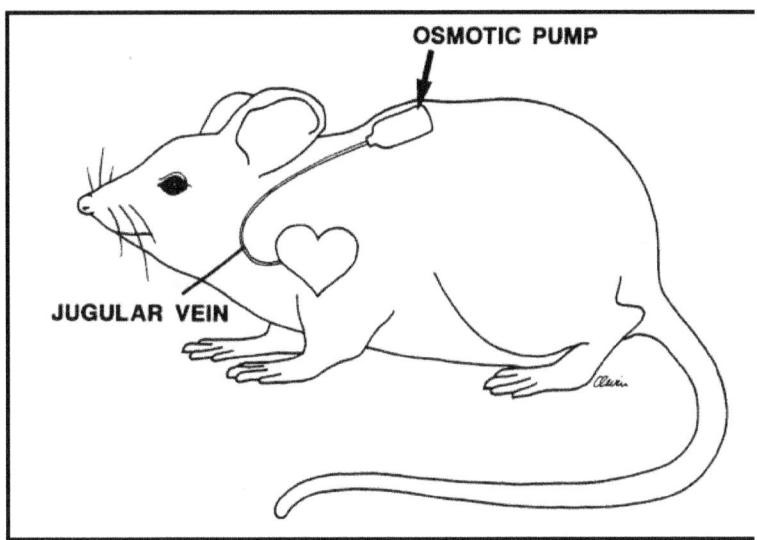

Figure 3. Cerulein model

Experimental design of the taurocholate time course study: Twenty-eight male Wistar rats, weighing 272-369 g, were randomly allocated to seven groups, as seen in Figure 4: One control group (n=4) and six taurocholate groups (n=4 in each). The control group was sham operated, i.e., they had a laparotomy followed by cannulation of the PBD, but with no duct infusion, and were sacrificed at zero hours. The rats in the taurocholate groups followed the same procedure, but were injected with taurocholate 3% (55.8 mmol/l) into the PBD. After 3, 6, 12, 24, 48 and 72 hours they had a new laparotomy under full anesthesia; the abdominal cavity was examined macroscopically to score the degree of AP, as described below. Hereafter, blood was drawn from the heart and the rats were sacrificed. The pancreas was quickly removed and was freed of fat and major lymph nodes and weighed.

Another four rats, weighing 264-281 g, were used to detect the maximum pressure during infusion of taurocholate. With the same procedure for induction of AP as described above, a water gauge was interposed between the infusion pump and the cannula. The pressure, expressed as cm H_2O, was monitored constantly. P_{sy}, the initial system pressures and $P_{max.}$, the maximum system pressure, were registered continuously during an infusion of the same volume as described above. As this experiment only served to determine the infusion pressure during induction of AP, no other variables were measured in these rats.

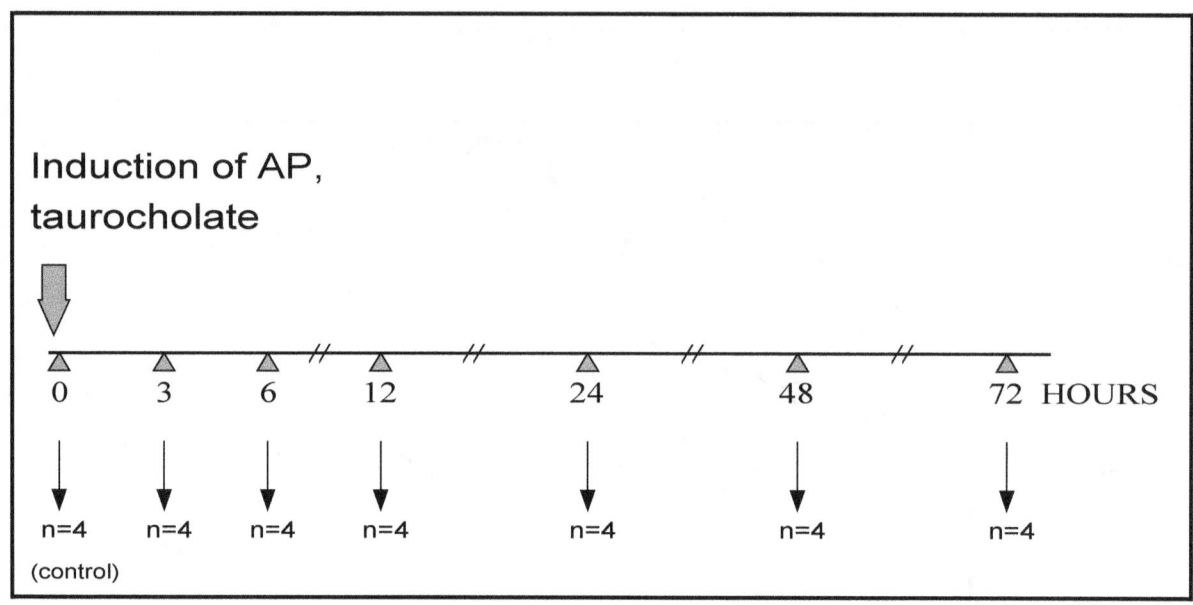

Figure 4. Design of the taurocholate time course study

Experimental design of the taurocholate dose response study: Twenty-eight male Wistar rats, weighing 261-298 g, were randomly allocated to seven groups: Six taurocholate groups were infused into the PBD with doses = 1, 2, 3, 4, 5 and 6 % (18,6 - 111,6 mmol/l, n=4 in each group) and one control group (0 %) was infused with sterile isotonic saline (n=4). Six hours after induction of AP, the animals were sacrificed by thoracotomy and exsanguination during anesthetic. Blood and pancreas were removed as described above. Laboratory determinations of α-amylase and lipase in plasma, peritoneal exudate, pancreatic wet weight and macroscopic scoring were performed for all the groups, and histological scoring was performed in dose groups 0, 1, 3 and 6 %, all as described below.

Experimental design of the cerulein time course study: Twenty-nine male Wistar rats, weighing 222 - 261 g, were randomly allocated to seven groups (See Figure 5): Control group (n=4) and cerulein groups, T= 3, 6, 12, 24, 48 and 72 hours (n=4 in each group). One rat from the 72 hour group was replaced before data processing due to misplacement of the catheter. The control group received pH adjusted physiologic saline via osmotic pumps and the rats were sacrificed after 6 hours of infusion. The cerulein group received cerulein dissolved in pH adjusted physiologic saline via osmotic pumps with an infusion rate of 10 µg/kg/h. The 48 and 72 hours groups received cerulein for only 24 hours in order to examine a possible spontaneous recovery. The animals had a laparotomy and were macroscopically examined at the given time points. Blood and pancreas were removed as described above. Finally, placement of the pump and the catheter was checked.

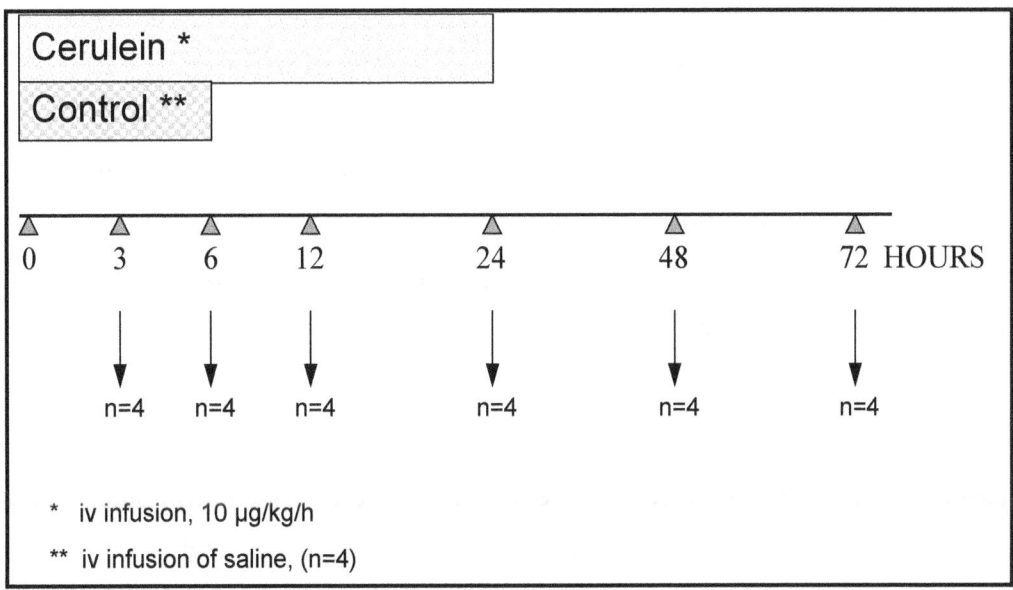

Figure 5. Design of the cerulein time course study

Peritoneal exudate and pancreatic wet weight: Peritoneal exudate was collected by absorbent cotton and weighed. The pancreatic wet weight was recorded and expressed as a ratio: pancreatic wet weight g/100 g body weight (BW).

Macroscopic scoring: Four categories were scored as we used a graduation from "none to severe": Extra pancreatic fat necroses (retroperitoneally and/or in the mesentery) (0-3), pancreatic edema (0-3), pancreatic hemorrhages (0-3) and pancreatic necrosis (0-3). The possible range of the total macroscopic score from each rat was from zero to 12.

Laboratory determinations: Blood was sampled from the heart and immediately kept at 0°C. The plasma was separated and stored at minus 20°C. Lipase and α-amylase activities were determined in plasma by two commercial kits (Lipase MPR1 and α-amylase EPS, Boehringer/Mannheim). The test principle for the lipase kit is the conversion of triolein by lipase to monoglyceride and oleic acid which leads to a decrease in turbidity measured in the UV range [114]. The test principle for the amylase kit is a two-step enzymatic colorimetric test with 4,6-ethylidene(G_7)-p-nitrophenyl(G_1)-α,D-maltoheptaoside as substrate [114b]. For these analyses we used a recording spectrophotometer (UV-2100, UV-VIS, Shimadzu Corp., Kyoto, Japan).

Handling of the pancreas: We pinned each pancreas on a cork plate, marked the duodenal part with Indian ink and fixed it for four days in formalin 10%. The pancreas was then embedded in 2% Genugel (Carrageenan, type X-0909, Copenhagen Pectin) and cut vertically into a series of slices with equal thickness. After that, each block was embedded in paraffin, cut in slices of 4 μm for light microscopy and stained with hematoxylin-eosin. A pathologist specialized in gastroenterology examined and graded two slices from the duodenal part and two from the splenic part of each pancreas with a blind observer design, i.e., no knowledge of the groups.

Histological scoring of the taurocholate model: We modified an established semi quantitative scoring system [115] to fit the changes we saw in this experimental model. The modification allowed the possibility of giving the score "none" for each of the histological patterns, permitting a scoring of the control group. As another modification, we simplified the grading of parenchymal necrosis, i.e., defining "focal necrosis" as involving parts of acini, "sublobular necrosis" as groups of necrotic acini surrounded by normal acini and "lobular necrosis" as involving whole necrotic lobuli. Histopathological patterns were graded as: edema (0-3), inflammatory infiltration (0-3), fat necrosis (0-7), parenchymal necrosis (0-7) and hemorrhage (0-7) (Table 8). Each slice could therefore obtain a possible range of a histological score from zero to 27. For each rat the total histological mean score of the four slices was then calculated.

Table 8. Histological scoring of the taurocholate model

Histological pattern and (score)	Assessment (score)
Edema	None (0)
	Mild (1)
	Moderate (2)
	Severe (3)
Inflammatory infiltration	None (0)
	Mild (1)
	Moderate (2)
	Severe (3)
Fat necrosis	None (0)
	< 2/section (3)
	3-5/section (5)
	> 5/section (7)
Parenchymal necrosis	None (0)
	Focal (3)
	And/or sublobular (5)
	And/or lobular (7)
Hemorrhages	None (0)
	Mild (3)
	Moderate (5)
	Severe (7)

Table 9. Histological scoring of the cerulein model

Histological pattern and (score)	Assessment
Interstitial edema	None (0)
	Mild (1)
	Moderate (2)
	Severe (3)
Inflammatory infiltration	None (0)
	Mild (1)
	Moderate (2)
	Severe (3)
Parenchymal necrosis (percentage of cells involved)	None (0)
	< 5 % (1)
	5- 25 % (2)
	25 - 50 % (3)
	> 50 % (4)
Vacuolization (percentage of cells involved)	None (0)
	< 5 % (1)
	5- 25 % (2)
	25 - 50 % (3)
	> 50 % (4)

Histological scoring of the cerulein model: We modified an established semi quantitative scoring system specifically intended for the changes seen in this model (Table 9) [116]. Histopathological patterns were graded as: Interstitial edema (0-3), Inflammatory infiltration (0-3), Parenchymal necrosis (0-4) and Vacuolization (0-4). Thus a possible range of the total histological score was from zero to 14. A whole organ total histological mean score was then calculated.

Statistics: The data was expressed as means $\pm$ SEM. Differences among the time groups were compared by the non-parametric one-way analysis of variances on the ranks, Kruskal-Wallis test for multiple groups. A multiple comparison of the different time groups versus controls was done according to Siegel [117]. Histological scores and plasma enzymes were compared using the non-parametric Spearman rank correlation method. In all instances, a $p < 0.05$ was considered statistically significant. Data handling and statistics were performed using the statistical software package STATISTICA, VER. 4.3, StatSoft Inc.

Ethics: The experimental procedures employed conform with the principles and practice of the Danish law regulating experiments on animals: *Lov om dyreforsøg* dated June 30, 1993. As a member of EU, Denmark is bound by Directive 86/609/EEC dated November 24, 1986.

Results

Taurocholate time course study: We observed no lethality in any of the different groups.

Plasma lipase and α-amylase activity levels increased significantly with time ($p < 0.05$, Kruskal Wallis), although we found different peak periods for the two enzyme activities. Figure 6 shows   that maximal lipase activity already occurred at six hours and was increased by 162 times above the control level with a return to near control values at 12 hours. Maximal α-amylase activity was found at 24 hours and was   12 times above the control level.

Peritoneal exudate increased significantly and reached a maximal value at 3 - 6 hours ($p < 0.05$, Figure 7).   At   24 - 72 hours, the   amount of peritoneal exudate had returned to a level not significantly different from that of the control group. Pancreatic wet weight ratios increased significantly ($p < 0.05$) to the highest level   in the 3 - 6 hour taurocholate groups. This was followed by a decline, and   in the 24 - 72 hour taurocholate groups the ratio was not significantly higher than in the control group.

Macroscopic scores were significantly higher in all taurocholate groups compared with controls ($p < 0.05$, data not shown).

The total mean histological scores continued to rise to a maximum at 24 - 72 hours, significantly higher compared with the control groups ($p < 0.05$, Figure 8).

The subgroups of the total mean histological score are presented in Figure 9: Edema increased significantly reaching a maximum at   24 - 72 hour   ($p < 0.05$). Inflammatory infiltration showed a significant   rise   reaching a peak level at 48 - 72 hours ($p < 0.05$). Fat necrosis was only found in the taurocholate   groups with significant high levels at 12 - 24 and 72 hours compared with the controls ($p < 0.05$). Parenchymal necrosis only occurred in the taurocholate groups with a steady increase towards 72 hours ($p < 0.05$). Hemorrhage was found in both the controls and the taurocholate groups with no significant difference between them. Additionally, we found signs of fibrotic degeneration in some histological slides in the taurocholate group at 48 hours whereas in all the slides in the taurocholate group at 72 hours (data not shown). The structural changes are shown in the Appendix, page 79.

The increase of plasma α-amylase activity during the first 24 hours correlated directly with the total mean histological score (Spearman's rank correlation coefficient = 0.50, p = 0.03). The increase of plasma lipase activity during the first 6 hours did not correlate with the total mean histological score (Spearman's rank correlation coefficient = 0.54, p = 0.07). As seen in Table 10, a subgroup analysis of histological scores showed that both plasma α-amylase and lipase activity correlated directly with edema, inflammatory infiltration and parenchymal necrosis, and did not correlate with fat necrosis and hemorrhages during the early stages of the disease. The total mean histological score did not correlate with plasma α-amylase or lipase activity when considering all the time groups (Spearman's rank correlation coefficients of 0.11 and 0.04, respectively).

Table 10. Subgroup analysis of histological scores versus plasma amylase (n=20) and lipase (n=12) activity: Spearman's rank correlation coefficient, (**=p<0.05).

	Edema	Inflammatory infiltration	Fat necrosis	Parenchymal necrosis	Hemorrhages
Amylase (0-24 h)	0.64**	0.76**	0.43	0.50**	0.41
Lipase (0-6 h)	0.65**	0.77**	0.40	0.77**	0.26

The bile infusion pressure, expressed as $P_{infus} = (P_{max}$, the maximum system pressure - P_{sy}, the initial system pressure), reached 20.6 ± 3.6 cm H_2O (± 95 % confidence interval: 9.2 - 32.0 cm H_2O).

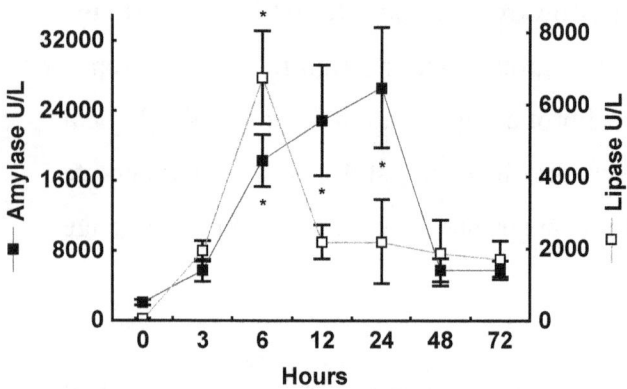

Figure 6. Taurocholate infusion, 3 %, time course study: Plasma lipase and amylase activity in the 0 - 72 hour groups (n=4 in each). Each point represents the mean ± SEM. *: p<0.05 compared with the 0 hour group (controls).

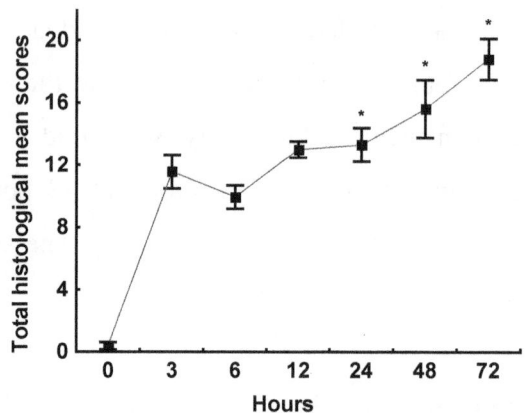

Figure 8. Taurocholate infusion, 3 %, time course study: The total histological mean score in the 0 - 72 hour groups (n=4 in each). Each point represents the mean ± SEM. *: p<0.05 compared with the 0 hour group (controls).

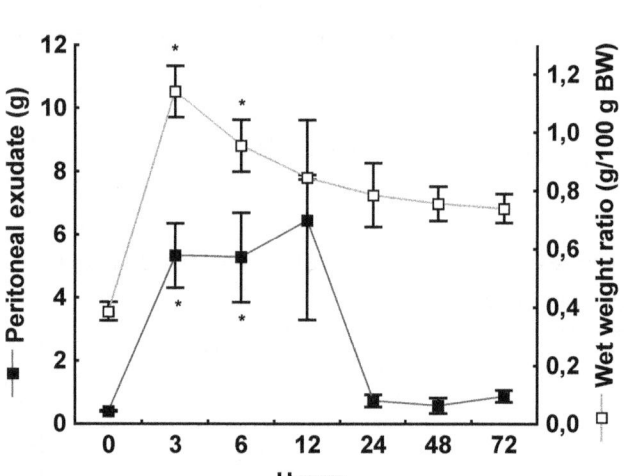

Figure 7. Taurocholate infusion, 3 %, time course study: Peritoneal exudate and pancreatic wet weight ratio in the 0 - 72 hour groups (n=4 in each). Each point represents the mean ± SEM. *: p<0.05 compared with the 0 hour group (controls).

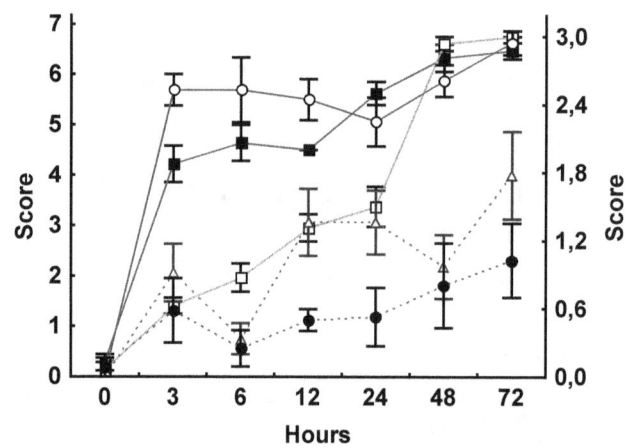

Figure 9. Taurocholate infusion, 3 %, time course study: Histological scores divided in subgroups: ■ Edema (0-3), □ Inflammation (0-3), △ Fat necrosis (0 -7), ○ Parenchymal necrosis (0-7), ● Hemorrhage (0 -7), in the 0 - 72 hour groups (n=4 in each). Each point represents the mean ± SEM.

Taurocholate dose response study: During the six hours of observation no lethality was found in any of the different groups.

Plasma α-amylase activity levels did not change with the different concentrations of taurocholate (p=0.29, Kruskal Wallis). The plasma lipase activity levels rose significantly in the different groups (p<0.05), reaching a nearly 4.8-fold plateau at a taurocholate dose of 4 %. In the 3 % taurocholate group a fall was seen (not significant) followed by a 2-fold rise in the 6 % group (p<0.05) (Figure 10).

Peritoneal exudate showed a significant increase (p<0.05) with a peak at 3 % taurocholate followed by a fall at 5% and an additional rise at 6% taurocholate (p<0.05). Pancreatic wet weight ratio rose to a significantly higher level in the 4 % taurocholate group (p<0.05) when compared with the 1 % taurocholate group (Figure 11). Macroscopic scores continued to rise in all the groups (p<0.05, Kruskal Wallis, data not shown).

The total mean histological scores were significantly different between the groups (p<0.05, Kruskal Wallis). The 0 % group was slightly, but not significantly higher than the 1 % taurocholate group and 0 % to 3 - 6 % taurocholate we found a significant increase (p<0.05) (Figure 12). The subgroups of the total mean histological score are presented in Figure 13: Edema, fat necrosis, inflammatory infiltration and hemorrhage showed no significantly difference between the groups. Parenchymal necrosis was significantly different between the groups (p<0.01, Kruskal Wallis), with a non significant fall from 0 - 1 % taurocholate followed by a continuous and significant (p<0.05) increase to a plateau at 3 - 6 % taurocholate. The structural changes are shown in the Appendix, page 80.

To test the reproducibility of this model, the results from the 6-hour group (3 % taurocholate dose) in the time-course study were compared with the results from the 3 % taurocholate -group of this study (6 hours). We found no significant difference regarding plasma α-amylase activity, peritoneal exudate, pancreatic wet weight ratio and the total histological mean score.

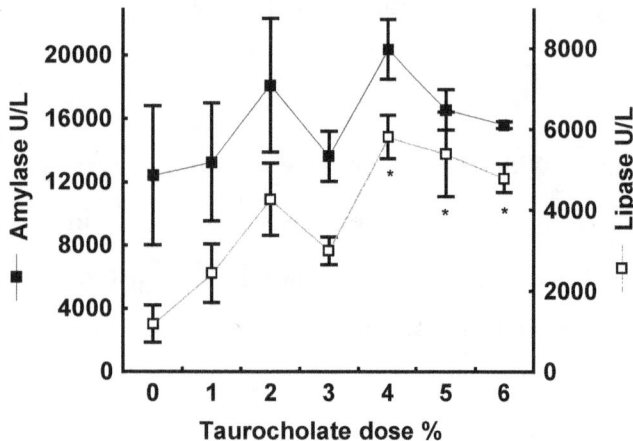

Figure 10. Taurocholate model, 6 hours dose-response study: Plasma lipase and amylase activity to increasing taurocholate doses (n=4 in each). Each point represents the mean ± SEM. *: p<0.05 compared with the 0 % group (controls).

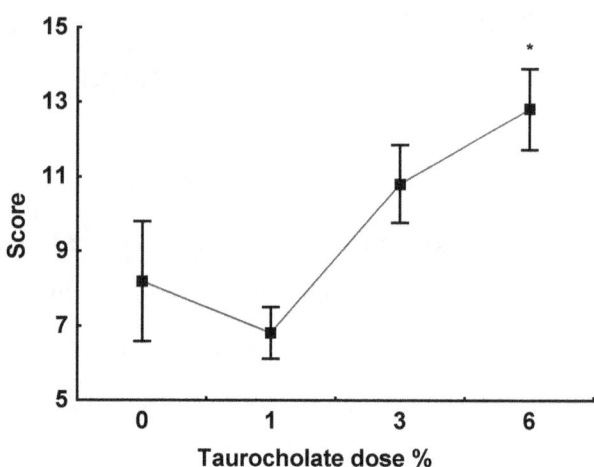

Figure 12. Taurocholate model, 6 hours dose-response study: The total histological mean score to increasing taurocholate doses (n=4 in each). Each point represents the mean ± SEM. *: p<0.05 compared with the 0 % group (controls).

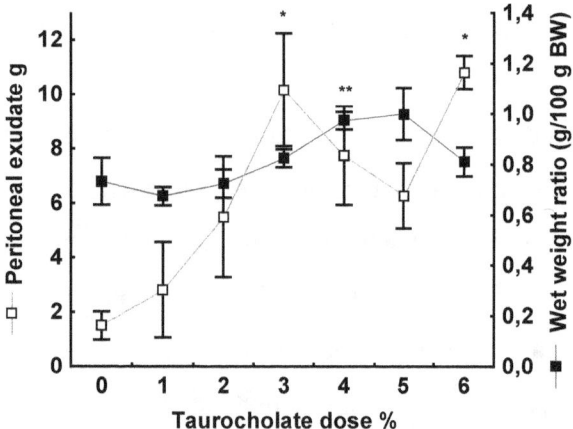

Figure 11. Taurocholate model, 6 hours dose-response study: Peritoneal exudate and pancreatic wet weight ratio to rising taurocholate doses (n=4 in each). Each point represents the mean ± SEM. *: p<0.05 compared with the 0 % group (controls). ** (wet weight ratio) p<0.05 compared with 1 % group.

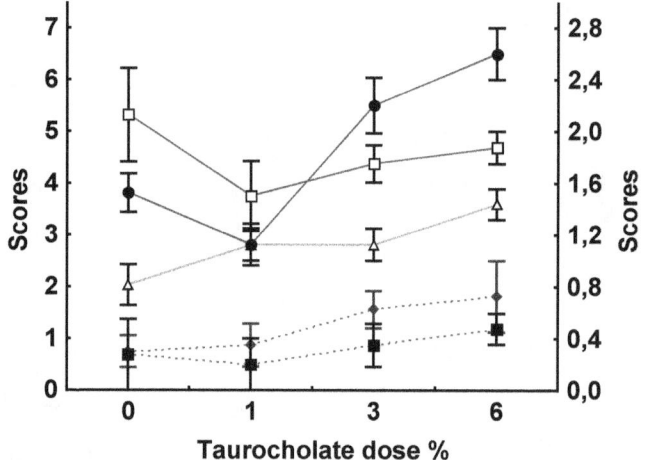

Figure 13. Taurocholate model, 6 hours dose-response study: Histological scores divided in sub-groups: □ Edema (0-3), △ Inflammation (0-3), ◆ Fat necrosis (0 -7), ● Parenchymal necrosis (0-7), ■ Hemorrhage (0 -7), to rising taurocholate doses (n=4 in each). Each point represents the mean ± SEM.

Cerulein time course study: We observed no lethality in any of the time groups. All pumps passed the quality control and delivered the expected amount of drug.

All animals responded macroscopically with maximal edema in the 3 - 24 hour groups and extra pancreatic fat necrosis appeared at 12 - 72 hours. We found no signs of pancreatic hemorrhage or necrosis in any of the groups (data not shown).

Plasma amylase and lipase activities were significantly different between the groups (p< 0.001, Kruskal Wallis) both peaking at 12 hours with a 32 fold rise for amylase and a 109 fold rise for lipase. At 24 hours, both enzyme activities had returned to values not significantly different from the controls (Figure 14).

The peritoneal exudate was significantly different between the groups (p<0.05, Kruskal Wallis), having a maximum at 12 hours. At 48 hours the peritoneal exudate had returned to control values. Pancreatic wet weight ratios peaked in the 6 - 12 hours groups all being significantly higher than the control group (p<0.05). At 24 hours the ratio had returned to a level not significantly different from the controls (Figure 15).

The total histological scores were significantly different between the groups (p<0.001, Kruskal Wallis) with a continuous rise until 24 - 72 hours (Figure 16).

The analysis of the subgroups in the total histological mean scores is shown in Figure 17: Edema showed to be an early phenomenon as the highest levels were seen already in the 3 hours group. This was followed by a decline towards 72 hours (p<0.05) not significantly higher than the controls. The same pattern was seen regarding vacuolization having the highest values at 6 - 12 hours followed by a fall to 72 hours being not significantly different from the controls. Necrosis and inflammatory infiltration showed another pattern. Scores of necrosis were significantly different between the time groups (p<0.001, Kruskal Wallis) with a continuous rise until 48 - 72 hours. Scores of inflammatory infiltration reached peak values at 48 hours (p<0.05 compared with the controls). The structural changes are shown in the Appendix, page 81.

The increase of plasma lipase and α-amylase activity during the first 12 hours correlated well with the total histological mean score (Spearman's rank correlation coefficients of 0.92 and 0.90, respectively, both p<0.001). As seen in Table 11, all the subgroups of the total histological scores, except one, correlated directly with plasma lipase and amylase activity. Edema did not significantly correlate with amylase.

Table 11. Subgroup analysis of histological scores versus plasma amylase and lipase activity (0-12 h) (n=16): Spearman's rank correlation coefficient, (**=p<0.05, # : p=0.051)

	Edema	Inflammatory infiltration	Parenchymal necrosis	Vacuolization
Amylase	0.49#	0.75**	0.88**	0.72**
Lipase	0.56**	0.73**	0.88**	0.73**

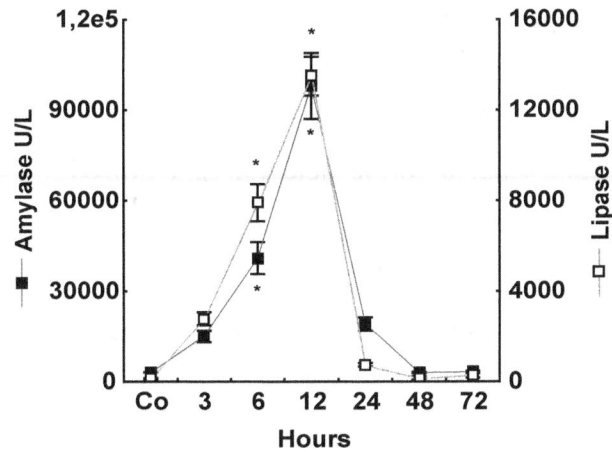

Figure 14. Cerulein model, time course study: Plasma lipase and amylase activity in different groups (n=4 in each). Each point represents the mean ± SEM. *: $p<0.05$ compared with the control group, Co.

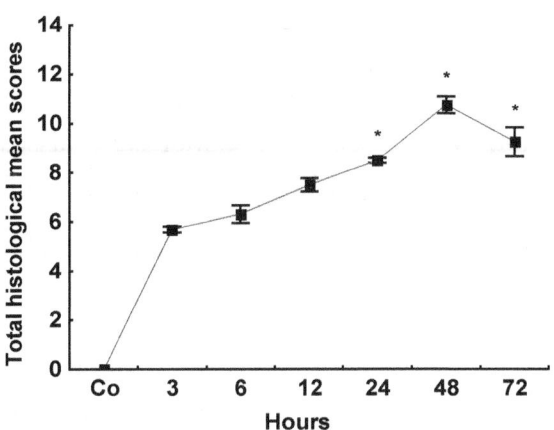

Figure 16. Cerulein model, time course study: The total histological mean score in the different groups (n=4 in each). Each point represents the mean ± SEM. *: $p<0.05$ compared with the control group, Co.

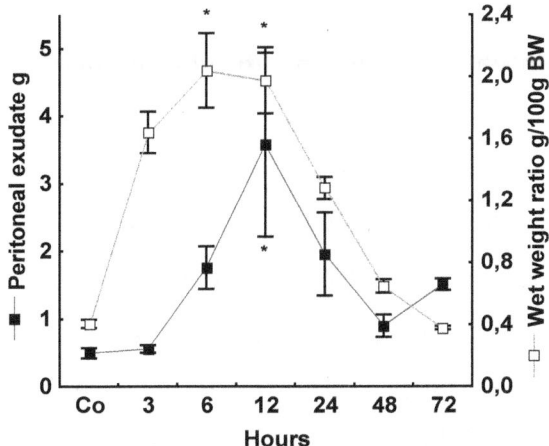

Figure 15. Cerulein model, time course study: Peritoneal exudate and pancreatic wet weight ratio in the different groups (n=4 in each). Each point represents the mean ± SEM. *: $p<0.05$ compared with the control group, Co.

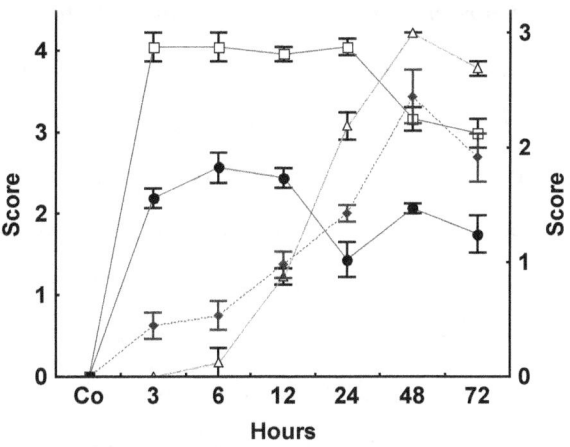

Figure 17. Cerulein model, time course study: Histological scores divided in subgroups: □ Edema (0-3), Δ Inflammation (0-3), ◆ Parenchymal necrosis (0-4), ● Vacuolisation (0-4) in the different groups (n=4 in each). Each point represents the mean ± SEM.

Part II: Involvement of ROS during early experimental AP

To investigate the possible involvement and importance of ROS in the two AP models in the rat, we conducted an initial study assessing the following: ascorbic acid (AA), oxidized ascorbic acid (DHAA), glutathione (GSH), oxidized glutathione (GSSG, only in pancreas) and lipid peroxidation measured as malondialdehyde (MDA) in plasma and in pancreatic tissue. Then, we conducted a full scale experiment on both models and measured the same variables. Additionally, we measured a marker of DNA-damage, 8-oxo-7.8-dihydro-2'-deoxyguanosine (8-oxodG), in the cerulein model.

Material and methods

Animals, anesthesia and analgesia: as described on page 19. The animals fasted 12 hours prior to induction of AP, with free access to water. After induction they had free access to both food and water.

Taurocholate model: As described on page 19 with an additional modification of the infusion method, a pressure controlled infusion pump was introduced. A commercial pump with the necessary specifications was not available, so we designed and tested our own pressure controlled infusion pump in order to optimize the taurocholate model. The pump consisted of an infusion pump controller (microprocessor controlled), an actuator unit carrying a 1 ml syringe, a connection to a Baxter Uniflow ® pressure transducer and a tube system connecting the syringe with the infusion catheter. Pump specifications and test sheet are presented in the Appendix on page 77 -78. The pump enabled us to infuse taurocholate into the PBD with a steady pressure below the physiologic pressure of about 28 cm H_2O. We used an infusion volume of 0.1 ml/kg BW, i.e., app. 250 µl per rat.

Cerulein model: As described on page 20.

Experimental design of the initial study: AP was induced in 12 male Wistar rats, weighing 215 - 245 g with the use of both models: 1) Taurocholate infusion of 3 % sodium taurocholate into the PBD (as described above) and 2) Cerulein i.v. infusion (10µg/kg/h). Three groups were considered: T=0, 1 and 2 hours, with n=2 in each group.   The controls, i.e., T=0, were sham operated   with no induction of AP.

Experimental design of the taurocholate study: 60 male Wistar rats, weighing   216 - 265 g, were randomly allocated to three groups: 1) **Controls**: sham operated 2) **Saline controls**: pressure controlled injection of saline into PBD and   3) **Taurocholate**: pressure controlled injection of 3 % taurocholate into the PBD. At 0, 2, 4, and 6 hours for the controls, and at 2, 4, and 6 hours for the saline controls and the taurocholate group, six rats from the each group were sacrificed after sampling of blood and tissue. All the above mentioned variables were assessed, except the marker of DNA oxidation, 8 oxodG.

Experimental design of the cerulein study: 43 male Wistar rats, weighing   232 - 275 g, were randomly allocated to two groups: 1) **Controls**: sham operated and i.v. infusion of saline, 2) **Cerulein**: infusion of cerulein i.v., 10 μg/kg/h). Due to pump failure in one rat from the cerulein group (the catheter fell off the pump), the rat was replaced by another before data processing. At 0, 4, 6   and 12 hours for the controls and at 4, 6   and 12 hours for the cerulein group, six rats from each group were sacrificed after sampling of blood and tissue, as described above. All the above mentioned variables were assessed including a marker of oxidative DNA damage, 8-oxodG. Due to lack of pancreatic tissue in   9 rats from the controls and in 3 rats from the cerulein group,   we could not assess 8-oxodG in these animals. For measuring   base line values of 8-oxodG, additionally 9 male Wistar rats, weighing 204 - 225 g,   were added to the control group (at 0 hours). We therefore assessed 8-oxodG in 39 rats; the control group consisted of 11, 4, 3 and 6 animals at the time points 0, 4, 6 and 12 hours, respectively, and the cerulein group consisted of 5, 4 and 6 animals at the time points 4, 6 and 12 hours, respectively.

Sample collection: EDTA- and heparin-treated blood was   drawn from the left ventricle of the heart in vacuum glass containers (Venoject ®). Then it was quickly centrifuged (10.000 x g, 1.5 min., 4 °C),   and plasma was derivatized according to the analyses described below and immediately stored at minus 70 °C. Pancreas was quickly removed, freed from fat and lymph nodes, rinsed in ice cold physiologic saline, blotted dry and freeze clamped in liquid nitrogen. The whole pancreas was then pulverized using a mortar and pestle on dry ice and immediately stored at minus 70 °C.

Laboratory determinations:

GSH/GSSG: EDTA-treated plasma was quickly acidified with 5-sulfosalicylic acid 10 % (w/v) and 0.3 mM diethylenetriamine-dipentacetic acid (DPTA), vortexed well and centrifuged (10.000 x g, 5 min., 4 °C). The supernatant was divided in two portions (one was derivatized with 2-vinylpyridine for GSSG measurement), and both portions were immediately stored at minus 70 °C. Pancreatic powder was homogenized in 5-sulfosalicylic acid 5 % (w/v) containing 0.3 mM DPTA using an iced teflon Potter-Elvehjem homogenizer (0.2 g tissue/ml). After centrifugation (10.000 x g, 10 min., 4 °C), the supernatant was collected, divided in two portions (one was derivatized with 2-vinylpyridine for GSSG measurement), and both were immediately stored at minus 70 °C. Plasma and pancreatic total GSH, i.e., GSH + GSSG, in GSH equivalents, and GSSG were determined spectrophotometrically (UV-2100, UV-VIS, Shimadzu Corp., Kyoto, Japan) using the 5,5'-dithiobis(2-nitrobenzoic acid), DTNB-GSSG reductase recycling assay for GSH, and for GSSG using 2-vinylpyridine for the GSSG determination [118].

AA/DHAA: EDTA-treated plasma was quickly stabilized with pre-cooled 10 % metaphosphoric acid (MPA), centrifuged (4000 x g, 10 min., 4 °C) and stored at minus 70 °C. Pancreatic powder was homogenized with a glass/glass homogenizer in pre-cooled 5 % MPA (0.05 g tissue/ml), centrifuged (4000 x g, 10 min., 4 °C) and stored at minus 70 °C. Ascorbic acid and dehydroascorbic acid were measured by HPLC [119].

MDA: EDTA-treated plasma was immediately stored at minus 70 °C. Pancreatic tissue was homogenized in ice cold 20 mM Tris-HCL buffer, pH 7.4 with a Potter-Elvehjem homogenizer (0.1 g tissue/ml), centrifuged (3000 x g, 10 min., 4 °C) and the supernatant was stored at minus 70 °C. MDA was measured spectrophotometrically using a commercial kit (Bioxytech® LPO-586, Oxis International, USA). A chromogenic agent 1-methyl-2 phenylindole, reacts with MDA to produce a stable chromophore with maximal absorbance at 586 nm (UV-2100, UV-VIS, Shimadzu Corp., Kyoto, Japan).

8-oxodG and deoxoguanosine (dG): Pancreatic tissue was homogenized in HEPES buffer (5 mM HEPES, 90 mM sucrose, 250 mM manitol, pH 7.4). 200 μl Homogenate was suspended in 1.8 ml ice-cold TE buffer (150 mM NaCl, 10 mM Tris, 10 mM Na_2EDTA, pH 8.0) and 200 µl of 10 % SDS was added. After vortexing for 30 sec., rotation for 15 min. and incubation in water bath (37 °C, 10 min.) the following were added: 200 µl 3 M sodium acetate (pH 5.2), 550 µl 5 M sodium perchlorate and 2 ml chloroform/isoamyl alcohol (24:1). After rotation in an extraction bench for 10 min., the supernatant (non-organic phase) was transferred to a tube and mixed gently with 2 x vol. of ice-cold 96 % ethanol. The DNA was allowed to precipitate at -20 °C overnight. The DNA precipitate was washed with 70 % ethanol, dried with a stream of nitrogen gas, solubilized in 200 µl 20 mM sodium acetate, pH 4.8, (37 °C, until dissolved). Thereafter it was incubated with Nuclease P1 (20 µl, 5 U/sample; Sigma, ST. Louis MO) for 30 min. Alkaline phosphatase (20 µl, 1 U/sample; Boehringer Mannheim, Germany) was then added and the DNA was digested to nucleoside level (37 °C, 60 min.). The samples were centrifuged (5200 x g, 4°C, 35 min.) in centrifuge filters (30 K MWCO, Whatman International, UK). Thereafter, the amount of 8-oxodG and dG were measured using HPLC with an electrochemical detector and UV as described in [120].

Plasma ∝-amylase and lipase: Heparin treated plasma was analyzed as described on page 23.

Pancreatic protein content: Protein in pancreas was measured by using the Lowry method with bovine serum albumin as standard [121].

Peritoneal exudate: As described on page 23.

Water content in lung, kidney and liver tissue: Immediately after sacrifice, the right lower lung lobe, the right lateral liver lobe and the right kidney were weighed (wet weight). After incubation at 70 °C for about one week (until steady weight was obtained) the dry weight was measured. Tissue water content was expressed as the ratio (wet weight - dry weight)/(wet weight).

Statistics: The data was expressed as means ± SEM. To approximate a normal distribution, a $\log_{10}$-transformation was performed. Homogeneity of variances was tested using Levene's test. Differences between the groups were tested using two-way analysis of variance (2-way-ANOVA). In all instances, a p-value less than 0.05 was considered statistically significant. All data handling and statistics were performed using the statistical software package STATISTICA 5.0 for Windows, StatSoft, Inc., 1996.

Ethics: The experimental procedures employed conform with the principles and practice of the Danish law regulating experiments on animals: *Lov om dyreforsøg* dated June 30, 1993. As a member of EU, Denmark is bound by Directive 86/609/EEC dated November 24, 1986.

Results

Initial study: In the taurocholate model, plasma and tissue content of total GSH decreased after 2 hours while an increase in tissue GSSG was observed. Plasma total AA decreased after 2 hours while tissue total AA was unchanged. High values of MDA both in plasma and in tissue was observed already after 1 hour (Table 12).

Table 12. Results from the initial study: Taurocholate and cerulein model. *: values near zero. #: only one value.

Hours	Plasma GSH µM	Tissue total-GSH nmol/mg protein	Tissue GSSG nmol/mg protein	Plasma total AA µM	Tissue total AA nmol/mg prot	Plasma MDA µM	Tissue MDA pmol/mg protein
Taurocholate model							
0 hours	28.6 - 29.5	7.22 #	0.61 - 0.84	79.6 - 89.8	2.59 - 5.01	0.16 - 0.23	*
1 hour	29.5 - 33.3	8.29 - 8.61	1.50 - 1.54	59.4 - 81.8	1.87 - 4.45	0.27 - 0.40	0 - 50.74
2 hours	25.0 - 25.4	4.83 - 8.36	1.28 - 1.29	50.6 - 56.2	2.29 - 2.68	0.27 - 0.38	0 - 5.2
Cerulein model							
0 hours	28.4 - 33.3	7.02 - 11.02	0.52 - 0.67	51.3 - 85.1	1.33 - 2.01	0.30 - 0.54	*
1 hour	40.3 - 89.1	9.43 - 9.49	0.74 - 1.01	59.2 - 106.0	2.03 - 2.08	0.62 - 0.73	*
2 hours	27.0 - 39.9	3.45 - 4.21	0.57 - 0.70	76.3 - 90.3	1.82 - 1.96	0.15 - 0.22	*

In the cerulein model, plasma total GSH was high in the 1 hour group, which might be due to hemolysis. Tissue GSH decreased after 2 hours while tissue GSSG slightly increased after 1 hour. Total AA in both plasma and tissue increased after 1 hour. Plasma MDA was slightly increased after 1 hour while all tissue MDA samples were below detection limit (Table 12).

38

Taurocholate study: All 60 rats survived the observation period. In the taurocholate group, all the animals developed macroscopic and enzymatic signs of AP. Due to surgical complications (perforation of the PBD and leakage from the duodenal puncture), two rats in the control group, one at 0 and one at 6 hours, were excluded before data processing.

Both plasma α-amylase and lipase activities were significantly higher in the taurocholate group compared with the two other groups ($p<0.001$, 2-way-ANOVA). An increase in levels over time was seen for both enzymes, and at 6 hours the amylase activity was 5.8-fold higher and lipase was 10-fold higher in the taurocholate group compared with the other two groups (Figure 18 and Figure 19). No significant difference was found in plasma lipase activity between the saline controls and the controls,, whereas plasma α-amylase activity was slightly higher in the saline group ($p=0.001$, 2-way-ANOVA). Another indicator of pancreatitis severity, peritoneal exudate, increased over time; at 4 hours, it was 2.1 fold and 6.7 fold higher in the taurocholate group compared with the control and the saline control groups, respectively ($p<0.001$, 2-way-ANOVA, Figure 20).

Protein content of pancreas decreased in the taurocholate group to 0.74 - 0.88 times that of the control group, which was significantly lower than the two other groups ($p<0.001$, 2-way-ANOVA, Figure 21). The water content of liver, kidney and lungs was not significantly different in the taurocholate group compared with the other two groups (data not shown).

Plasma GSH in the taurocholate group decreased significantly during the observation time of six hours: 0.66 times that of controls and 0.78 times that of saline controls ($p=0.04$, 2-way-ANOVA, Figure 22). GSSG in pancreas, as a % of total GSH, was not significantly higher in the taurocholate group compared with the other groups ($p=0.06$, 2-way-ANOVA, Figure 23) or when compared with the control group alone ($p=0.07$, 2-way-ANOVA). Total GSH in the pancreas, when related to wet weight, was significantly lower in the taurocholate group ($p<0.001$, 2-way-ANOVA, Figure 24); at 4 hours, the taurocholate group was 0.49 and 0.65 times that of controls and saline controls, respectively. When correction is made for edema by expressing the total GSH in pancreas per mg of protein, the taurocholate group was significantly lower than the control group ($p=0.004$, 2-way-ANOVA, Figure 25) but not significantly different when compared with the saline control group ($p=0.08$, 2-way-ANOVA);

at two hours the total GSH in pancreas in the taurocholate group was 0.74 and 0.70 times that of controls and saline controls, respectively.

Total plasma AA was not significantly different in the taurocholate group compared with the other two groups ($p=0.14$, 2-way-ANOVA, Figure 26). Plasma DHAA, as a % of total AA, was not significantly different between the groups ($p=0.34$, 2-way-ANOVA) and the overall mean was not significantly different from zero (-0.37, -0.94 - 0.21: mean, 95 % confidence interval, data not shown). Pancreatic total AA, when related to wet weight, was significantly lower in the taurocholate group, compared with the other two groups ($p=0.011$, 2-way-ANOVA, Figure 27); at 6 hours the taurocholate group was 0.76 and 0.75 times that of controls and saline controls, respectively. But when related to mg of protein, there was no significant difference between the taurocholate group and the other two groups ($p=0.76$, 2-way-ANOVA, data not shown). DHAA in pancreas, as a % of total AA, was not significantly different between the groups ($p= 0.07$, 2-way-ANOVA) and the over all mean was not significantly different from zero (0.68, -1.45 - 0.090: mean, 95 % confidence interval, data not shown).

MDA in plasma did not differ significantly in the taurocholate group compared with the other two groups ($p=0.08$, 2-way-ANOVA, Figure 28). MDA in pancreatic tissue, when related to wet weight, was not significantly different between the taurocholate and the control groups ($p=0.45$, 2-way-ANOVA). When related to mg of protein, there was a significant difference in the pancreatitis group compared with the other two groups ($p=0.003$, 2-way-ANOVA, Figure 29), but no difference was found when comparing the taurocholate group with the controls ($p=0.40$, 2-way-ANOVA).

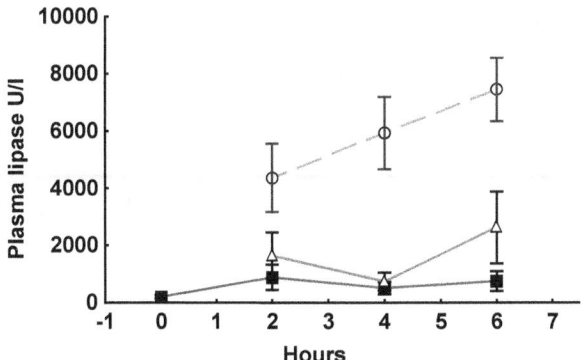

Figure 18. Taurocholate study: Plasma lipase activity U/l (p<0.001, 2-way-ANOVA).

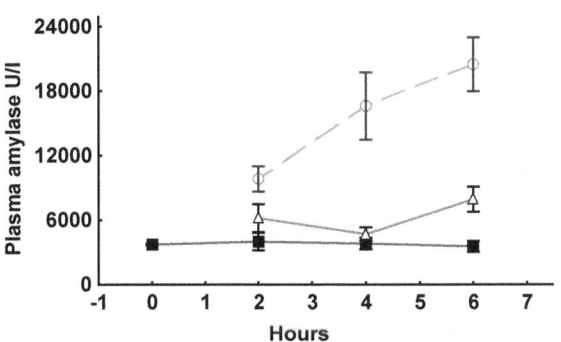

Figure 19. Taurocholate study: Plasma amylase activity in U/l, (p<0.001, 2-way-ANOVA).

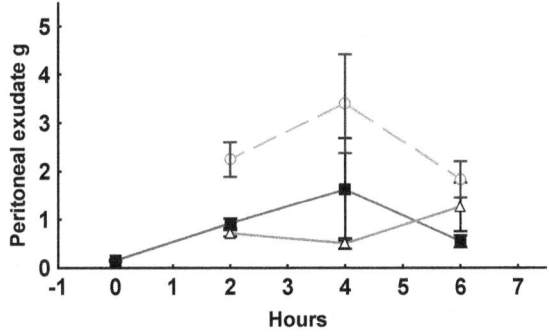

Figure 20. Taurocholate study: Peritoneal exudate in g, (p<0.001, 2-way-ANOVA).

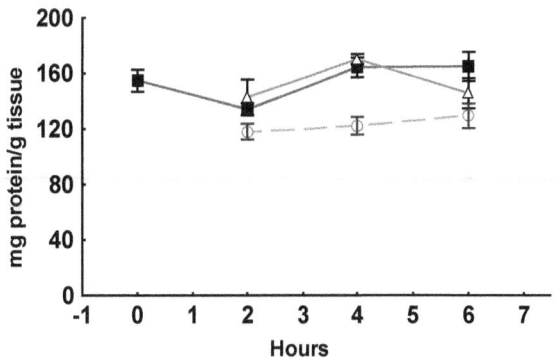

Figure 21.Taurocholate study: Pancreatic protein content in mg/mg tissue wet weight (p<0.001, 2-way-ANOVA).

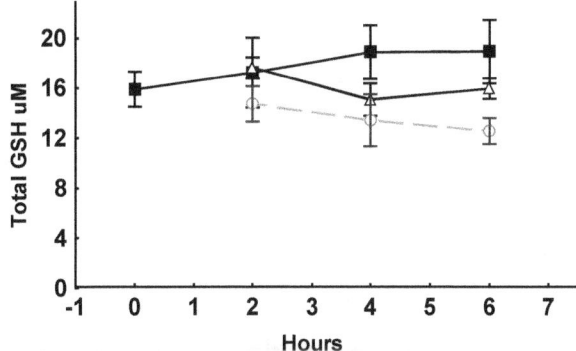

Figure 22. Taurocholate study: Plasma total GSH in μM, (p=0.036, 2-way-ANOVA).

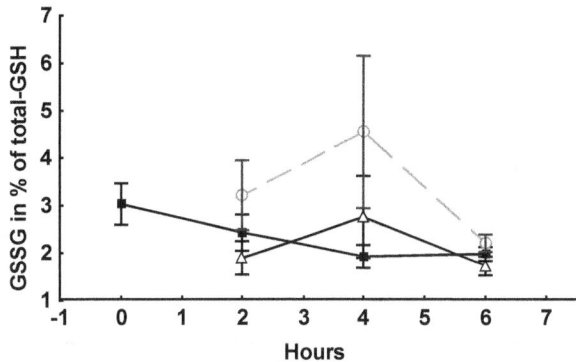

Figure 23. Taurocholate study: Pancreas GSSG as a % of total GSH, (p=0.06, 2-way-ANOVA).

Figure legends: ■ **Controls** △ **Saline controls** ○ **Taurocholate**
Each time point (n=5-6) is described by mean ± SEM

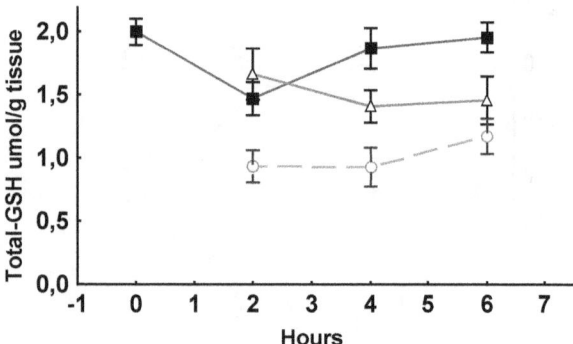

Figure 24. Taurocholate study: Pancreatic total GSH in μmol/g tissue wet weight, (p<0.001, 2-way-ANOVA).

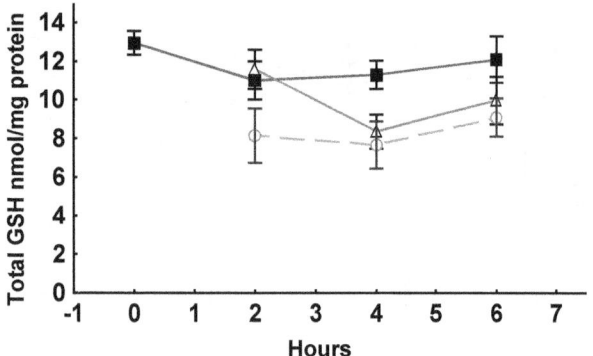

Figure 25. Taurocholate study: Pancreatic total GSH in nmol/mg protein, (p=0.004, taurocholate vs. controls, p=0.08, taurocholate vs. saline controls 2-way-ANOVA).

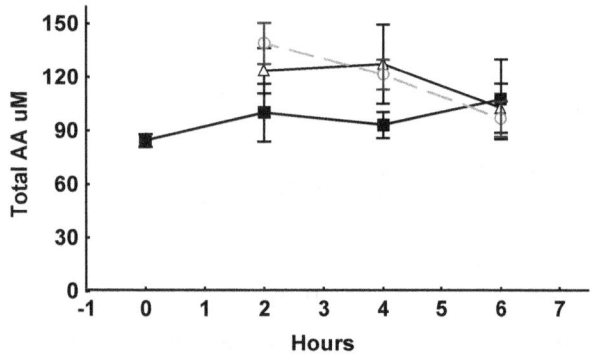

Figure 26. Taurocholate study: Plasma total AA in μM, (p=0.14, 2-way-ANOVA).

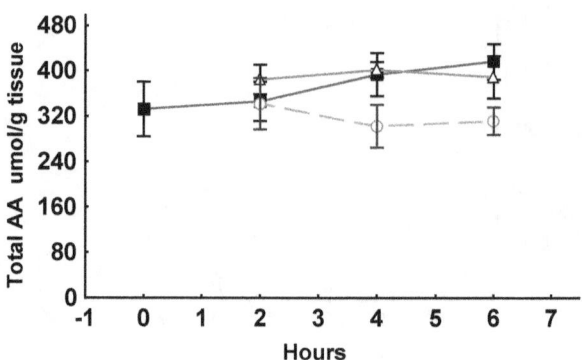

Figure 27. Taurocholate study: Pancreatic total AA in nmol/g tissue wet weight, (p=0.011, 2-way-ANOVA).

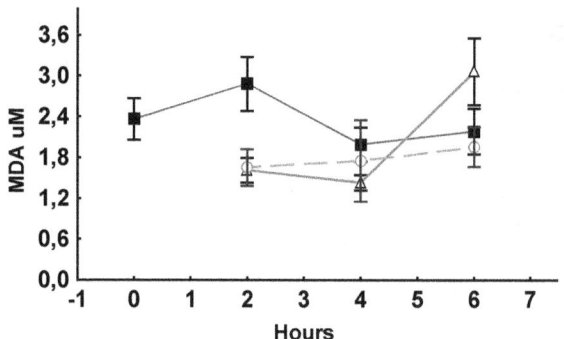

Figure 28. Taurocholate study: Plasma MDA in μM, (p=0.08, 2-way-ANOVA).

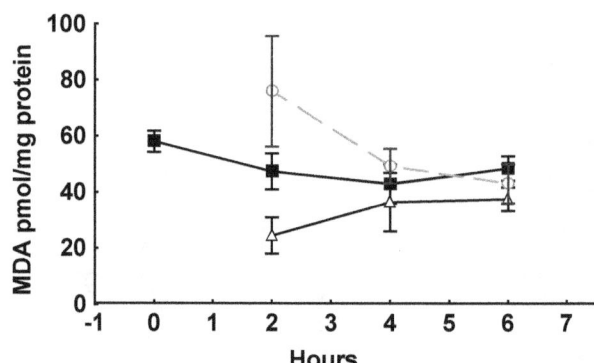

Figure 29. Taurocholate study: Pancreatic MDA in pmol/mg protein, (p=0.003, 2-way-ANOVA).

Figure legends: ■ **Controls** Δ **Saline controls** ○ **Taurocholate**
Each time point (n=5-6) is described by mean ± SEM

Cerulein study: All 43 rats survived the observation period, one rat was excluded as described on page 35. In the cerulein group, all the rats developed macroscopic and enzymatic signs of AP.

Both enzyme α-amylase and lipase activities in plasma increased over time and were significantly higher in the cerulein group compared with the control group ($p < 0.0001$, 2-way-ANOVA). At 12 hours, α-amylase and lipase were 27 and 139 times higher, respectively, in the cerulein group compared with the control group (Figure 30 and Figure 31). Peritoneal exudate increased over time in the cerulein group and at 12 hours a 4.7-fold increase was observed. The amount of peritoneal exudate was significantly higher in the cerulein group compared with the control group ($p < 0.0001$, 2-way-ANOVA, Figure 32).

Pancreatic protein content decreased in the cerulein group to 0.56 times that of the control group ($p < 0.0001$, 2-way-ANOVA, Figure 33). The water content of the liver and the lungs was significantly lower in the cerulein group versus the control group ($p < 0.01$, 2-way-ANOVA, data not shown), whereas no statistical difference was found for the water content of the kidneys (data not shown).

Plasma total GSH was slightly lower, but not significantly different in the cerulein group compared with the control group ($p = 0.06$, 2-way-ANOVA, Figure 34). Pancreas-GSSG, in a % of total GSH, increased in the cerulein group to a 1.9 times higher level at 4 hours and continued the increase to a 3.4 times higher level at 12 hours, compared with the control group ($p < 0.0001$, 2-way-ANOVA, Figure 35). Total GSH in pancreatic tissue when related to wet weight, was significantly lower in the cerulein group compared with the control group ($p < 0.0001$, 2-way-ANOVA, Figure 36). When related to mg of protein, the cerulein group was still significantly lower than the control group ($p < 0.0001$, 2-way-ANOVA, Figure 37); 0.54 times and 0.71 times that of controls at 4 and 6 hours, respectively.

Plasma total AA was significantly higher in the cerulein group as compared with the controls ($p < 0.0001$, 2-way-ANOVA, Figure 38); at 12 hours, the controls were 0.26 times the level of the cerulein group. P-DHAA, as a % of total AA, was not significantly different between the two groups ($p = 0.86$, 2-way-ANOVA) with an over all mean below zero (-3.0, -4.1 - (-1.9): mean, 95 % confidence interval, data not shown). Total AA in pancreas, when related to wet weight, was significantly lower in the cerulein group compared with the control group (p<0.0001, 2-way-ANOVA, Figure 39). However, when related to mg of protein, no significant difference was seen between the cerulein group and the control group (p=0.87, 2-way-ANOVA, data not shown). DHAA in pancreas, as a % of total AA, was not significantly higher in the cerulein group, compared with the control group (p=0.13, 2-way-ANOVA) and the overall mean was not significantly different from zero (0.011, -1.08 -1.10: mean , 95 % confidence interval, data not shown).

In plasma, the levels of MDA was not significantly different from the levels in the control group (p=0.91,   2-way-ANOVA, Figure 40). Pancreatic levels of MDA, when related to wet weight and mg of protein, were significantly lower in the cerulein group compared with the control group (p<0.05, 2-way-ANOVA, Figure 41).

The 8-oxodG/dG ratio in pancreatic tissue was not significantly different in the cerulein group compared with the control group (p=0.93, 2-way-ANOVA, data not shown).

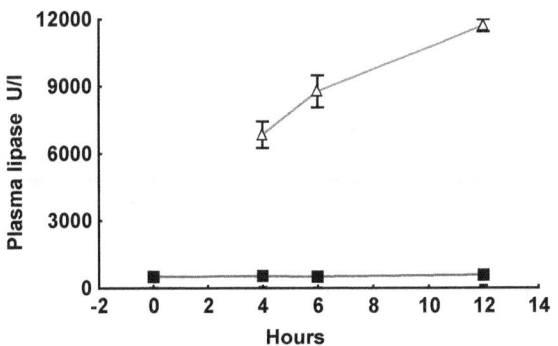

Figure 30. Cerulein study: Plasma lipase activity in U/l, μM, (p<0.0001, 2-way-ANOVA).

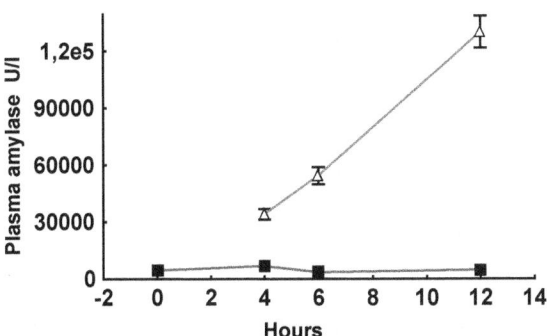

Figure 31. Cerulein study: Plasma amylase activity in U/l, (p<0.0001, 2-way-ANOVA).

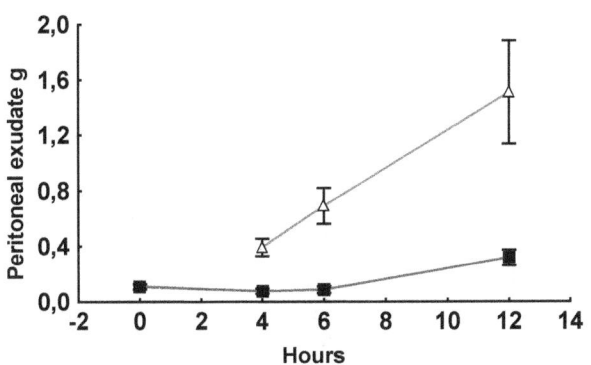

Figure 32. Cerulein study: Peritoneal exudate in g, (p<0.0001, 2-way-ANOVA).

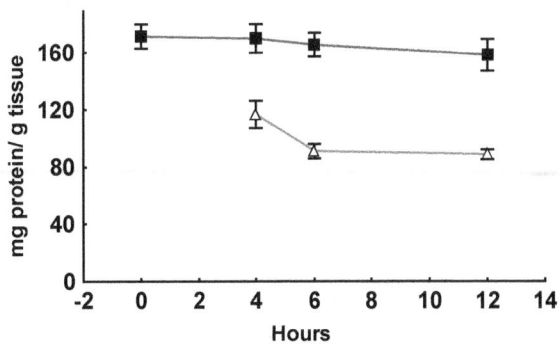

Figure 33. Cerulein study: Pancreatic protein content in mg/g tissue wet weight, (p<0.0001, 2-way-ANOVA).

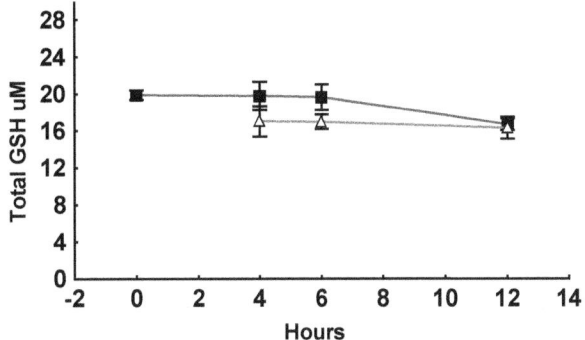

Figure 34. Cerulein study: Plasma total GSH in μM, (p=0.06, 2-way-ANOVA).

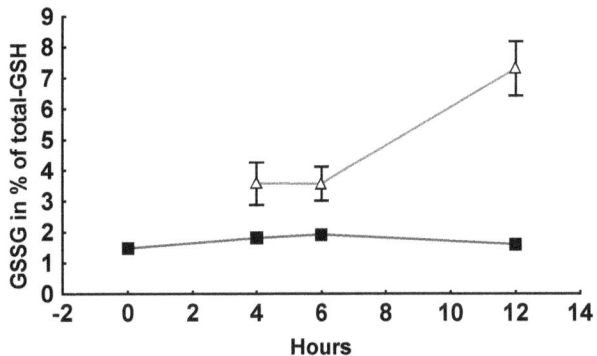

Figure 35. Cerulein study: Pancreatic GSSG in a % of total GSH, (p<0.0001, 2-way-ANOVA).

Figure legends: ■ Control   Δ Cerulein.
Each time point (n=6) is described by mean ± SEM

45

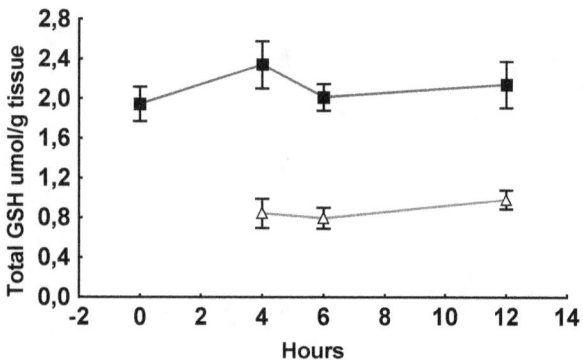

Figure 36. Cerulein study: Pancreatic total GSH in μmol/g tissue wet weight, (p<0.0001, 2-way-ANOVA).

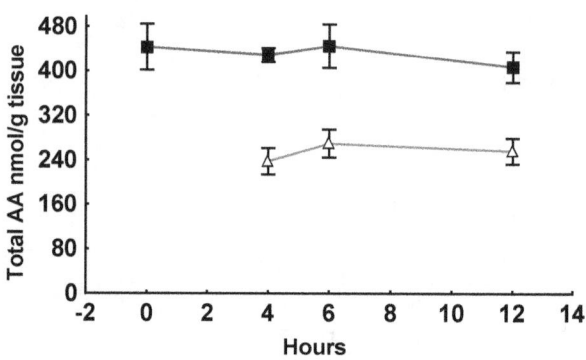

Figure 39. Cerulein study: Pancreatic total AA in nmol/g tissue wet weight, (p<0.0001, 2-way-ANOVA).

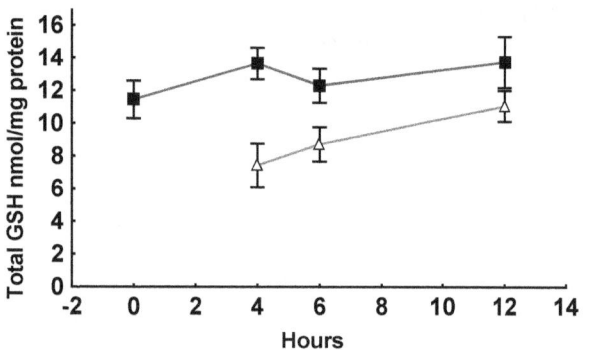

Figure 37. Cerulein study: Pancreatic total GSH in nmol/mg protein, (p<0.0001, 2-way-ANOVA).

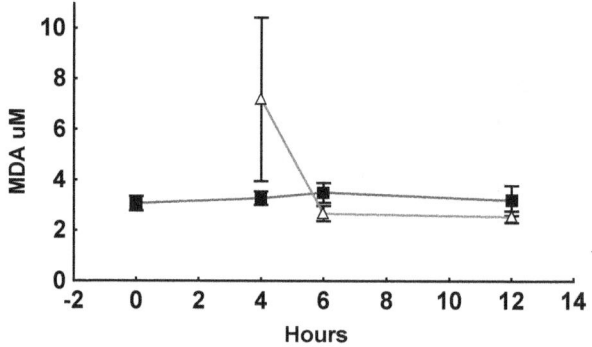

Figure 40. Cerulein study: Plasma MDA in μM, (p=0.91, 2-way-ANOVA).

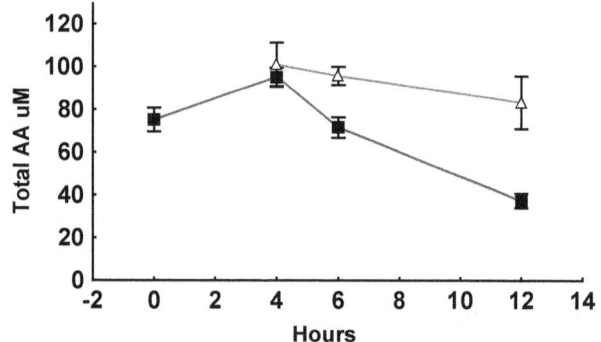

Figure 38. Cerulein study: Plasma total AA in μM, (p<0.0001, 2-way-ANOVA).

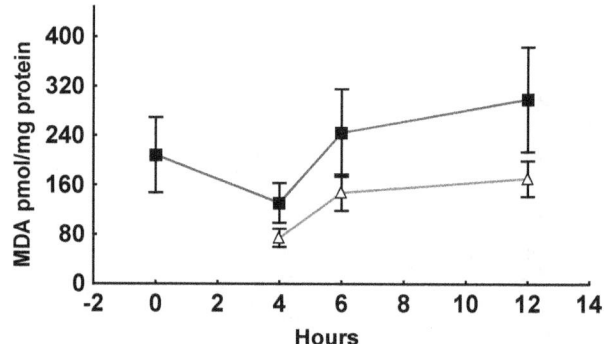

Figure 41. Cerulein study: Pancreatic MDA in pmol/mg protein, (p<0.05, 2-way-ANOVA).

Figure legends: ■ Control △ Cerulein.
Each time point (n=6) is described by mean ± SEM

Discussion

This study was conducted in two parts: *Part I* was a characterization of two AP models in rat undertaken in order to understand the development of the induced changes and to investigate any resemblance to the human disease. *Part II* was an attempt to test our hypothesis as to whether an early ROS involvement was likely in experimental AP, and if so, what importance it could have to the disease. This division into two parts is maintained in the following discussion.

Part I: Characterization of the two models

Taurocholate model - time course study: The outcome and the lethality of taurocholate induced experimental AP can be adjusted to the same outcome and lethality as in human AP, by changing the composition and volume of the infusion liquid [122]. The concentration of the injected sodium taurocholate can vary from 0.25 - 10% using volumes from 0.1 - 0.3 ml/100 g body weight. The lethality found in one study with 3, 4.5 and 5% sodium taurocholate, was 23.5, 71.5 and 100% respectively within a period of 72 hours [14]. As lethality is a non-specific and unethical variable, we intentionally wanted it minimized. We found no lethality with 3% taurocholate, and this may be explained by longer infusion time of the same volume and the choice of a more gentle anaesthesia. Another important factor to the lethality of this model might be the use of the analgesic buprenorphine as it seems very efficient in minimizing postoperative pain. Furthermore, buprenorphine does not interfere with the course of this experimental model in rat [111] .

Armstrong et al. emphasized the importance of controlled infusion pressure and controlled volume in this model [123]. He concluded that infusion of a small volume of 50 μl and an infusion pressure of 20 cm H_2O gave leakage from the pancreatic ducts via intercellular clefts and at 50 cm H_2O via duct rupture. Therefore, experiments of this kind were claimed to be relevant only when using a volume less than 50 μl with careful consideration given to the pressure [123]. The average duct pressure recorded during infusion of 550 μl taurocholate in the pancreatic duct in rat, at which rupture of the pancreatic duct occurred, was 112 cm H_2O [124]. Such a high pressure certainly exceeds the physiological secretory pressure. We used volumes of about 250 µl per infusion and found no infusion pressures exceeding 50 cm H_2O. Our model showed mean infusion pressures around 20 cm H_2O. Nevertheless, the optimal application would naturally be a pressure controlled infusion system with a pre-set maximum infusion pressure around 28 cm H_2O, i.e., the physiological secretory pressure found in rats [125]. Following this, we modified this model by introducing a pressure controlled infusion pump, as described on page 34.

Macroscopic evaluation correlated well with the histological changes scored with a semi quantitative scoring system when applied on three AP models in rat [115]. In our study, the macroscopic evaluation was performed by the same person responsible for the induction of the AP in the rats, therefore being highly biased. Thus, we only used the macroscopic evaluation as a quality control of the AP model.

Histopathological scoring is considered a standard variable in experimental AP [9, 13] yet there is no consensus onto which classification systems should be preferred. The modified scoring system we used was reliable to detect the early changes seen in the light microscopic slides (see examples in the Appendix page 79). These changes resemble the histological changes seen in human severe AP such as sub-lobular and lobular coagulative necroses, inflammatory infiltrates and interstitial hemorrhage [126]. Additionally, we found "plugging" of small vessels by leukocytes as seen in human AP [126]. The scoring system was not designed to detect late changes such as fibrosis, as we found in all the rats 72 hours after induction of AP. We chose to study the early events of AP and thus we found no late complications, as in late human AP, such as pancreatic pseudocysts or pancreatic abscesses. Aho et al. found small pancreatic abscesses after 72 hours in rats surviving injection of 3 - 4.5 % taurocholate into the PBD [14]. But we did not find any other reports of such complications in the literature dealing with long term studies on the taurocholate model in rat.

Bile-induced AP develops morphologically in two stages [127]. Initially, an acute detergent effect of the bile salt is followed by the histological changes of hemorrhage, edema and necrosis. The acute stage occurs within 15 minutes of induction of AP, at which time histological changes such as pancreatic edema and necrosis is found [14]. Later, the involvement of activated proteolytic enzymes will lead to autodigestion thus resulting in more hemorrhage, edema and necrosis. In our study we could confirm such a two-stage activity with a very rapid formation of edema and necrosis followed by inflammation, fat necrosis and more necrosis at 24 hours and so on.

Peritoneal exudate accumulation is frequently seen in patients with AP [128], and in our study this was an early indicator of the severity of the disease. Peritoneal exudate was used as a variable in an intervention study, where treatment with scavengers significantly reduced the production of peritoneal exudate [97]. As a measure of the pancreatic edema, a ratio between the pancreatic wet weight and the body weight has been used [78], and in one study the ratio was significantly well correlated with the degree of histological edema [123]. Measuring the water content in the rat pancreas by drainage is possible [14], however, this would exclude a histological analysis of the whole gland.

Activity levels of plasma lipase and α-amylase can be used to monitor the progression of AP [9]. In our study both indicator enzymes increased initially. Plasma lipase activity increased to a higher maximum faster than plasma amylase activity. Plasma amylase activity declined to control levels later than the lipase activity. Similar results were seen in human AP, where serum lipase increased to a far higher level than serum amylase, but afterwards, both enzymes returned to a normal range at about the same time [129]. It was suggested that serum lipase had a shorter $T_{1/2}$ than serum amylase [129]. In fact, this was verified experimentally in rats and dogs [130]. We found peritoneal exudate and pancreatic wet weight ratio to be early markers of AP. The pancreatic water content was significantly increased as early as 15 minutes after induction of taurocholate pancreatitis in rat, which partly supports our data [131].

We found severe histological damage of the pancreas even when the values of amylase, lipase and peritoneal exudate had nearly become normal. Schmidt et al. found, that serum amylase correlated well only with pancreatic edema and peripancreatic fat necroses, parameters not considered to be indices of severity in pancreatitis; the usual indices of severe pancreatitis - acinar necrosis, hemorrhage, intra lobular inflammation and perivascular infiltrate - correlated poorly with the levels of serum amylase [132]. Our study supports these findings, when considering the total histological scores for the period 0 - 72 hours. However, in the acute phase from 0 - 24 hours, the serum amylase activity levels could be used as an index of severity in our experimental model. Similarly in human AP levels of serum amylase, when compared with the clinical severity, showed a bell-shaped curve; low values indicated either no injury or a severe pancreatic injury while high levels were related to intermediate pancreatic injury [133].

Taurocholate model - dose-response study: The chosen time course of 6 hours seemed to be appropriate, because it avoided death as an end point. No lethality was observed before 6 hours in a study that used 3-5 % taurocholate and the same volumes as in our study [14]. When a three times larger infusion volume was used, the lethality rates at 6 hours were 25 and 50 % for 3 and 5 % taurocholate, respectively [134].

In our study, even injection of sterile isotonic saline in the controls resulted in elevated plasma levels of pancreatic enzymes and histological signs of pancreatitis. Infusion of small volumes (50 μl) of sterile isotonic saline under increasing pressures resulted in rises in amylase levels, in macroscopic and in histological edema [123]. As controls, sham operation without any duct infusion was described by Aho et al. [131]. Others have, as controls, used duct infusion of isotonic saline with the same volume and infusion speed as the experimental taurocholate group [135]. Thus, besides control of volume, pressure and concentration of the infusion liquid, an optimal study design should contain two control groups: One sham operated group and another control group which had injection of saline into the PBD. Again our findings supported the need of a pressure controlled infusion in this model to avoid or at least to control any pressure induced pancreatic damage, as mentioned above.

With increasing concentrations of taurocholate in the infusion liquid, we observed a dose-response relationship on the plasma lipase levels, the macroscopic and total histological values. We did not find a dose-response relationship on the plasma amylase activity level. The most likely explanation for this, could be high initial values in the 0 % group (controls) due to pressure induced damage, that would "flatten" the dose-response curve. Likewise, we found high initial values of lipase, macroscopic indicators and histological scores in the 0 % group The taurocholate dose being in the "middle" of the dose-effect curve, was 3%. Thus, the relevant dose for the optimal study design seemed to be 3 % taurocholate, since it would allow detection of both increases or decreases in the assessed variables. Furthermore, with 3 % taurocholate death as an endpoint was avoided with a time course of 6 hours.

The total histological mean score showed a dose-effect relationship, and the predominant histological subgroup factor was parenchymal necrosis. In the taurocholate time course study, parenchymal necrosis reached a maximum by 3 hours, while the other subgroups reached a maximum at later times. Thus, the most sensitive early histological variable seemed to be the measuring of the parenchymal necrosis. In this study we used a modified semi-quantitative scoring [115], but a quantitative tool would be even more sensitive. This could be accomplished by measuring the area of necrosis with a computer guided morphometric analysis [136], or even better by measuring relative volumes of necrosis by modern stereologic methods.

Taurocholate induced AP in rats has similarities with the human AP such as morphology, function and complications [122]. This model attempts to mimic gallstone induced pancreatitis in humans where three mechanisms of etiology have been suggested as viable: 1) The "common channel theory" [5], i.e., an impacted gall stone at the duodenal papilla results in bile regurgitation into the pancreatic duct. 2) The "obstruction theory" [137], i.e., a stone obstructing the pancreatic duct leading to pancreatic secretion against an obstacle. 3) The "duodenal reflux theory", i.e., a damaged sphincter of Oddi due to a passed gall stone would allow duodenal contents to reflux into the pancreatic duct [138]. As the pressure in the human pancreatic duct exceeded the pressure in the common bile duct [139], and as perfusion of sterile bile through the pancreatic duct in animals under physiological pressure did not result in any cellular damage [140], these theories are questionable. Thus, it is doubtful whether the etiology of the taurocholate model in fact is the same as in the clinical situation.

Cerulein model - time course study: Cerulein, a decapeptide isolated from the skin of the frog Hyla caerula, is a CCK-analogue. With intravenous infusion of cerulein in maximal physiological doses, i.e., the maximal secretory dose (0.25 µg/kg/h in rat), the secretory activity and protein synthesis increased and a degranulation of the pancreas with a 90 % reduction of the enzyme stores within 24 hours was seen [113]. The increased protein synthesis returned to normal after 48 - 72 hours [113]. No degenerative changes occured in the exocrine pancreas and no rise of plasma enzymes (amylase and lipase) activity levels with the use of up to 0.5 µg/kg/h cerulein was found [110, 113].

When the cerulein dose was increased to 20 times that of maximal secretory doses, i.e., supramaximal stimulation, the result was pancreatic damage with edema, elevation of pancreatic enzymes in plasma and morphological changes characteristic of acute pancreatitis [23]. While the pancreatic juice output was increased with maximal physiologic stimulation (0.25 µg/kg/h of cerulein), it was reduced to near zero values after few hours of supramaximal stimulation (5 µg/kg/h of cerulein) [110]. Dose-response studies on rats showed maximal values of pancreatitis indicator enzymes in plasma (a 4-fold rise for amylase and a 200-fold rise for lipase) at cerulein doses of 5 - 7.5 µg/kg/h after 3 hours of i.v. infusion [110] or 20 - 50 µg/kg/4h by subcutaneous injections [116].

The mechanism of how cerulein in supramaximal doses results in AP, is still unclear. Saluja et al. showed that cerulein interaction with low affinity CCK-receptors on the acinar cell surface mediated an inhibition of enzyme secretion from the pancreas, and suggested that this could lead to AP [141]. The exocytosis of the zymogen granules at the luminal part of the acinar cell plasma membrane was blocked and a premature fusion of condensing vacuoles and secretory granules led to formation of large cytoplasmic vacuoles [23]. The vacuoles then fused with the basal and lateral plasma membrane and emptied their content into the extracellular space which led to an activation of the enzymes and to an autodigestion of the pancreas [23, 142]. Another theory is the one of "co-localization" of digestive zymogens with lysosomal enzymes; the normal separation of digestive zymogens and lysosomal enzymes was disturbed so they remained in the same compartment, which resulted in intracellular activation of digestive enzymes by lysosomal hydrolases [143].

Cerulein induced AP in rats is fully reversible and no lethality has ever been reported [144]. After three days of high connective tissue turnover, an increased mitotic activity in the pancreas was found [145]. Pancreatic tissue regenerated completely, and within 14 days after induction of cerulein induced AP both morphological and biochemical changes had disappeared [116, 146]. As we only followed the animals 48 hours after cessation of cerulein infusion, the time span was not long enough to see a total pancreatic regeneration. If rats were subjected to severe stress, such as water immersion, the cerulein induced pancreatitis was aggravated from edematous to hemorrhagic AP [147]. To minimize stress from immobilization of the animals, we chose the use of mini-osmotic pumps, and as a result of this, we found no signs of stress induced pancreatic hemorrhage.

In accordance with [23, 116] we found that plasma amylase activities continued to increase until 12 hours with a return to control values at 24 hours. Plasma lipase activity followed the same trend. As we infused cerulein for 24 hours and saw plasma enzyme levels decreasing 12 hours earlier, this could mean that the continuous hyperstimulation emptied the enzyme stores of the pancreas. In fact, Tani et al. showed that a marked reduction of enzymes in the pancreas took place in a cerulein rat model, and that this depletion persisted for seven days [116]. We found that peritoneal exudate and pancreatic wet weight ratio followed the same pattern and time course as the indicator enzymes. The wet weight ratio was an early severity indicator and was in accordance with our results on the histological edema.

The histological scoring system we modified was sufficient to detect the early changes in the cerulein model: Edema and vacuolization were the earliest morphological changes observed [110, 116]. This corresponded well with our results with maximal scores in the 3 hour group for both the histological variables. Ultra structural studies on pancreatic acinar cells in human AP showed similar vacuolization as large autophagic vacuoles containing cell organelles [148]. Inflammatory infiltration was noted nine hours after initiation of cerulein induced pancreatitis in mice [58], and we found manifest inflammatory infiltration at 12 hours. The initiation time and the extent of acinar cell necrosis have been reported very differently. Tani et al. found less than 5 % of the acinar cells necrotic at any time point, beginning at 4 hours after start of infusion [116]. Others found necrosis after 12 hours involving up to 60 % of the acinar cells [75], while in our study we found 30 - 40 % necrosis at 12 hours with a drop to less than 25 % necrosis at 72 hours. Both inflammatory infiltration and necrosis in the pancreas are seen in human AP [126]. We found no fibrosis and no complications such as pancreatic cysts or abscesses. But after 72 hours, we found all the rats had "tubular" complexes in the histological slides of the pancreas. These duct tubular structures has also been reported in human AP [149]. We found a good correlation between the indicator enzymes and the histological subgroup scores during the initial 12 hours. This corresponds well with the findings of Tani et al., who stimulated   with cerulein 80 μg/kg s.c. over a period of 12 hours and found the histological alterations near control values after 24 hours [116]. However, when we stimulated with cerulein for 24 hours, with a slightly higher cerulein dose, 10 μg/kg/h i.v., the histological scores were high even 48 hours after cessation of the hyperstimulation. This suggested that the histological damage in this model depended not only on the cerulein dose, but also on the stimulation time.

The etiology   of cerulein induced AP is probably not the same as that of human AP since only a few human cases are due to supramaximal stimulation of the acinar cells: Accidental exposure to insecticides or to rare scorpion venom   [150-152]. Grönroos et al. suggested a theory of "the cholinergic hypothesis of alcoholic pancreatitis"; chronic alcohol intake could change the control of the exocrine pancreatic secretion through interference with the cholinergic and pancreozymin pathway   [153]. This theory would increase the importance of experimental hyperstimulation models, such as the cerulein model, but whether this   theory is relevant in alcohol induced human AP, is still unclear. Nevertheless, the cerulein rat model shared other similarities, apart from etiology, with the human AP such as: structural changes of the acinar cells   [154], local biochemical changes in the pancreas   [155] and multi-organ involvement such as adult respiratory distress syndrome (ARDS)   [60].

Part II: The involvement of ROS

Initial study: Taking the small sample size in consideration, the following could be concluded: The   assays   we used were reliable and the scavenger levels were as expected. Technically, sampling of tissue and plasma was possible. GSH measurement   in plasma was very sensitive to hemolysis, but this could be controlled by using vacuum glass containers instead of plastic syringes, thus we optimized this procedure. For both models, the tissue MDA values were around 0. To determine if this was due to a malfunction of the assay, pancreatic tissue from control animals was incubated with ascorbic acid and ferrous sulphate (a radical inducing Fenton-system). This resulted in a linear increase in pancreatic MDA from 100 % initially to 196 (192-204.) % after 1 hour, and   to 306 (302-310) % after 2 hours (expressed as mean % of controls, min. - max.). DHAA values both in tissue and in plasma were all around 0 (data not shown).

The taurocholate model showed a slightly earlier time course compared with the cerulein model, with earlier depletion of scavenger pools and earlier detection of MDA in plasma. This was consistent with the results from the characterization of the models. Therefore, a relevant time course for a full scale study was 0 - 6 hours for the taurocholate model and 0 - 12 hours for the cerulein model.

Full scale study: In tissue injury, such as during AP, an overproduction of ROS has been suggested to be a contributor to further cellular damage: Initial injury → ROS formation → antioxidant depletion → oxidative cell damage [27, 156]. Thus, a potential involvement of ROS in experimental acute pancreatitis could be assessed in three experimental designs, as described on page 13: by the direct measurement of ROS in-vivo, by the treatment of the animals with specific scavengers thus blocking the development on to cellular damage and finally by the measurement of endogenous scavengers. As direct measurements of ROS in-vivo has until recently been impossible, the direct assessment of antioxidants in the relevant compartments and markers of oxidative cellular damage seems at present to be the most indicative way to investigate a potential ROS involvement in diseases. Therefore this approach was chosen for our study.

The direct approach by measuring specific ROS with the use of ESR-techniques is encumbered by technical problems, especially when dealing with in-vivo models. The short lived radicals, such as $^\bullet$OH, are difficult to observe with ESR-techniques. However, spin-trapping agents can be added to create spin-adducts with a longer half life and thus ROS become easier to detect [10]. But many of these spin-trapping agents are in themselves toxic and consequently may not be suitable for in-vivo experiments [157]. The only study using ESR on experimental AP in mice induced by a CDE-diet indicated a production of the hydroxyl radical after 12 - 24 hours by detection of an increase in a OH-adduct [68].

An alternative method for direct detection of ROS in-vivo is chemiluminescence, where the emission of light due to electron transfer in chemical reactions is used as an index of ROS activity [10]. But the specificity of this method has been questioned; factors like pH, temperature and albumin may interfere with the light emission [10]. In experimental AP, taurocholate, cerulein and closed duodenal loop models all showed an early increase in chemiluminescence after 0.25, 0.33 and 6 hours, respectively [69-71].

The most popular approach has been the indirect evidence obtained from interventional studies, with the use of scavengers against ROS. Mostly by pretreatment (before induction of AP) with scavengers such as SOD, catalase and allopurinol, the histology and pancreatic enzyme levels in blood were assessed. If these scavengers were specific, with the sole biological action as scavengers and no other biological effects, their efficacy would be indicative of an involvement of ROS. In at least two studies, with cerulein and CDE-diet induced AP in mice and rats, catalase diminished the markers of tissue injury and improved survival both when active, but also when inactivated by boiling. The latter result was explained as an nonspecific protein effect [79, 86]. Unfortunately, this problem of specificity has not been considered in other studies. The cellular availability of enzymatic scavengers, such as SOD, has been questioned, since externally infused SOD does not enter the cells [99]. Finally, in spite of the numerous studies on treatment with scavengers, no dose-response relationship has been performed on experimental AP.

The results of these scavenger studies has appeared somewhat confusing and seemed to depend on the kind of AP induced. In three studies on ex-vivo perfused dog pancreas, SOD, catalase and allopurinol treatment led to less tissue injury and to lower pancreatic enzyme levels in plasma [12, 66]. Cerulein induced AP in rats and mice treated with SOD, catalase and allopurinol, showed positive results on tissue damage and on pancreatic enzyme levels in nearly all the reported experiments [73, 74, 76, 81]. In three cerulein studies, a positive effect was found on pancreatic edema but no effect on pancreatic enzyme activities in blood [75, 79, 80]. Generally, the results from the taurocholate model have been negative [80, 82, 83, 85]. SOD and catalase treatment led, in one study, to less edema but had no effect on pancreatic enzyme activity levels in plasma [84]. However, the opposite effect has also been found with catalase and SOD showing no effect on edema but a positive effect on necrosis and on pancreatic enzyme levels [81]. In the severe CDE-pancreatitis, contradictory results have been reported. When treating with allopurinol or catalase, or allopurinol and DMSO no positive influence was found on either tissue damage or pancreatic enzymes in blood [85, 86]. The same scavengers with comparable concentrations caused less edema and a lower level of pancreatic enzymes in blood [80].

Our main finding was an early depletion of GSH in pancreas in both models. The most severe depletion was seen in the cerulein model at the first time point (4 hours): Pancreatic total GSH was 43 % lower than in the control group when related to protein content. This was followed by an increase in the pancreatic GSSG/GSH-ratio from about 1 % in the controls to 7 % in the cerulein group after 12 hours. In the taurocholate model, we found a depletion of pancreatic GSH of 26 % at the earliest time point of 2 hours, followed by a borderline, but not significant, increase of pancreatic GSSG/GSH ratio at 4 hours. A significant increase in the latter result might have been detected with a larger sample size. In plasma, GSH was slightly depleted in the taurocholate model by 24 % but no depletion was detected in the cerulein model. Luthen et al. found, in cerulein induced AP in rat, a 72 % decrease in pancreatic total GSH after 4 hours, when related to pancreatic wet weight [94]. When based on protein content, the decrease could however be calculated from the presented data to 37 %, which was in the range of our results. But Luthen et al. found no increase in pancreatic GSSG [94]. During the same time course, two cerulein studies in mice showed a 83 % and a 76 % depletion of pancreatic total GSH, both relating the concentrations to wet tissue weight [96, 158]. As could be seen from our characterization of both models, a severe pancreatic edema took place over time. This was also indicated by a lowered protein concentration in pancreatic tissue in our ROS study. Accordingly, a dilution of almost any substance measured in the pancreas takes place. Indeed, a more relevant presentation of endogenous antioxidant concentrations would be one related to dry matter, such as protein or DNA content. Thus the above reported impressive data relating to tissue wet weight, should be interpreted with care. In taurocholate induced AP, the above reported changes seemed to be the same, but occurred within a shorter time frame. GSH rapidly decreased by 52 % at 0.5 hours followed by an early increase in GSSG/GSH-ratio in pancreas from 2.7-13.8 %, control group versus AP group [97]. This data was confirmed by another study with the same taurocholate model [98]. The experimental design in our taurocholate study did not allow a conclusion on changes in GSH in less than 2 hours after induction.

Theoretically, the observed depletion of pancreatic GSH could be caused by several factors, such as consumption of GSH while neutralising ROS or by mechanisms affecting the synthesis of GSH in the pancreatic cells: decreased energy supply or lack of precursor amino acids and enzymes. As we observed an increase in the oxidized form of glutathione, GSSG, in the cerulein model, an involvement of ROS was possible. In the taurocholate model, this theory seemed less probable. In both models a severe depletion of pancreatic ATP has been found following the exact time course of the GSH depletion [94, 97]. This impaired energy supply has been proposed to slow down the cellular GSH synthesis [94]. Only one study has looked at the precursor amino acid, cysteine, in cerulein induced AP in mice, and a pancreatic cysteine depletion was parallel with a GSH depletion [158]. But a drug induced increase of intracellular cysteine content did not avoid the cerulein induced GSH depletion [158]. Thus, it is still unclear what causes the observed GSH depletion during experimental AP and further research is needed for clarification.

To our knowledge, no previous studies have measured reduced and oxidized AA during experimental AP. We found no decrease in AA that could be ascribed to the changes due to the induction of AP, and furthermore we found no increase in DHAA. In two studies on cerulein and CDE pancreatitis in mice, the beneficial effect of a synthetic scavenger made from ascorbic acid, 2-octadeacylascorbic acid, was investigated. This ascorbic like scavenger had a strong therapeutic effect on both tissue damage [87] and on survival [78], but other beneficial effects than the antioxidant effect could have been possible.

The actual importance of depletion of the antioxidants AA and GSH in the cells, has been the issue of many studies. By experimentally depleting tissue GSH by administration of buthionine sulfoximine in mice, a corresponding decrease in tissue AA in lung and kidney followed by an increase in DHAA occurred within a few hours [159]. Interestingly, AA in liver increased rapidly within the first few hours of GSH depletion in mice, which suggested the liver to be the major site of ascorbate synthesis in this species [159]. When liver GSH in mice was depleted by three different GSH depleting agents, liver necrosis accompanied by increased lipid peroxidation only occurred when GSH was severely depleted, i.e., depletion of 85 - 90 % of control values [160]. Severe depletion of GSH in pancreas in adult mice did not cause any morphological damage in the pancreas [161]. Depletion of total GSH in rat lung tissue by 50 % did not lead to structural changes of the lungs, not even when exposed to lethal hyperoxia [162]. In-vitro studies with human umbilical vein endothelial cells depleted more than 90 % of their GSH, showed that ascorbate, both intra- and extracellularly, protected against the toxicity of exposure to nitrogen dioxide [163]. These results suggested, that a minor GSH depletion per se did not lead to oxidative cellular damage especially when AA levels are unchanged as seen in both our models. Thus it remains unclear what the significance of a minor depletion of pancreatic GSH during AP could be.

As markers of local oxidative cellular damage, we used MDA in both models and 8-oxodG/dG in the cerulein model. A less specific marker of remote organ damage was the change in the water content in the lung, liver and kidney. We found no relevant increased levels of MDA in the cerulein model. In the taurocholate model, pancreatic MDA was significantly higher at 2 hours when comparing the taurocholate group with the saline controls, but no difference was found when comparing with the controls. In both models, injection of isotonic saline seemed to decrease the MDA levels in the pancreas, when related to protein content. However, the cause of this effect remains unexplained. In other studies measuring markers of lipid peroxidation, such as malondialdehyde, conjugated dienes and thiobarbituric acid reactive substances, all showed a significant increase after 3 - 6 hours [75, 92, 93, 95]. The MDA content in rat pancreas has been measured to be between 0.4 - 1.1 nmol/ mg protein [97] and in plasma between 0.34 - 4.0 nmol/ml (normal and sick, respectively) [164]. With a detection limit of the MDA assay used in our study of 0.1 nmol/ml, the abnormal values in plasma and both normal and abnormal values in pancreas were within detection range of this assay.

DNA damage due to ROS, here measured as the 8-oxodG/dG ratio, has to our knowledge not previously been assessed in experimental AP. 8-oxodG has been used as a marker of early oxidative stress after ischemia/reperfusion injury in liver and small intestine transplantation in pigs. As early as 1 - 3 hours after reperfusion, the levels of 8-oxodG in urine were significantly increased when compared with the control group [165]. Chemically induced oxidative stress by administration of potassium bromate, in-vivo, showed formation of 8-oxodG in the kidneys and with the same time course showed increased lipid peroxidation [166, 167]. Lipid peroxidation products were shown to induce 8-oxodG in isolated DNA in an in-vitro study [168]. In our study we found no elevation in pancreatic 8-oxodG/dG ratio even 12 hours after induction of AP with cerulein thus indicating no oxidative DNA damage exceeding the repair capacity of the cells. GSH and AA have shown to be protective factors against DNA oxidation in rat kidney [167]. In our study, the remaining pancreatic GSH and AA might have been such a protective factor to the DNA.

8-oxodG has been suggested as a biomarker of oxidative DNA damage [52] and oxidatively damaged DNA may lead to an increased cancer risk in man [52]. In a recent case-control study, chronic pancreatitis was related to the increased incidence of pancreatic cancer in humans, whereas no relation was found to AP [169]. However, in another follow-up study, patients with more than one discharge diagnosis of AP had an increased risk of pancreatic cancer [170]. Even though an acute DNA oxidation does not seem to occur in the early phase of this cerulein model, a long term experiment is still needed in order to disclose whether a potential link between AP and pancreatic cancer exists due to oxidative damage to DNA.

ROS formation in experimental AP has been suggested as a contributor to the development of extrapancreatic organ failure in lungs, liver and kidney. In humans, multiple organ failure occurs in about 24 % of the patients with severe AP [171]. A ROS mediated injury to the endothelial barrier has been suggested as the pathogenic mechanism to AP induced multiple organ failure [172, 66]. In taurocholate induced pancreatitis, a significant increase in tissue water content was found in spleen, pancreas, kidneys, liver, lungs and heart [83]. In the same study, radio labelled albumin given i.v., leaked from blood to the tissue, also indicating an increased endothelial barrier permeability. Interestingly, this increased permeability was inhibited by the antioxidant and glutathione precursor N-acetyl-L-cysteine [83]. In neither of our AP-models, did we find any increase in water content in the liver, lung and kidney. This might, however, be due to a short observation time. Long term studies measuring both reduced and oxidized antioxidants in liver, lung and kidney, including markers of oxidative cell damage, would clarify the involvement of ROS in multiple organ failure due to AP.

Conclusions and perspectives

Model characterization: We found that in a direct model of acute pancreatitis, infusion of 3% sodium taurocholate into the pancreatic duct induced an initial increase in plasma lipase and α-amylase activity and in peritoneal exudate followed by a return to near control levels after 72 hours, whereas the total histological score and the pancreatic wet weight ratio remained high during this period. With increasing doses of taurocholate and an observation time of 6 hours, we saw a rise in plasma lipase activity, in macroscopic and histological variables.

In an indirect model of acute pancreatitis, supramaximal stimulation with cerulein induced an initial increase in plasma lipase and α-amylase activities, peritoneal exudate and pancreatic wet weight ratio with a return to control values within 48-72 hours, whereas the total histological score continued to increase.

This study showed together with the available literature, that both the taurocholate and the cerulein model in rat were reproducible models for induction of morphological and biochemical changes that are seen in the early stages of human AP. The taurocholate model was rapid and mimicked a severe necrotizing AP with graduated lethality. Conversely, the cerulein model was delayed and mimicked an edematous type of fully reversible AP with no lethality at all. Since one animal model does not cover the diversity of the human disease, the two models should be conducted together when investigating the pathophysiology of AP.

ROS study: We found that pressure controlled infusion of taurocholate into the pancreatobiliary duct induced acute pancreatitis in rats with the observed changes: A decrease in pancreatic protein content, no increased water content in liver, lungs or kidneys, a 24 % depletion of plasma total GSH and a 26 % depletion of pancreatic total GSH but no increase in pancreatic GSSG/GSH-ratio, no depletion of total AA and no increase in DHAA in neither plasma nor pancreas. These events were followed by a minor increase in pancreatic MDA but not in plasma MDA.

Supramaximal stimulation with cerulein, induced AP in rats with the following changes: A decrease in pancreatic protein content, no change of water content in liver, lungs or kidneys, no change of plasma total GSH, an early 46 % depletion of total GSH in pancreas, followed by an increase in pancreatic GSSG/GSH-ratio, no depletion of AA and no increase in DHAA in neither plasma nor pancreas. Finally, we found no increase in neither plasma nor pancreatic MDA levels and no increase in pancreatic 8-oxodG/dG ratio.

The early and moderate depletion of pancreatic glutathione in both models followed by an increase in the oxidized form of this antioxidant in the cerulein model were less than expected in our hypothesis. We fount neither an expected decrease in another important reducing agent, ascorbic acid, nor an increase in the oxidized ascorbic acid in any of the AP models. Furthermore, markers of oxidative damage to lipids and DNA, did not increase as we initially hypothesized. Our findings suggest, that the production and presence of ROS per se does not seem to have a major involvement in the initial steps of these two experimental models. Thus, ROS seems to be a result, rather than the course to acute pancreatitis.

This study on the involvement of ROS in experimental AP leaves several questions to be answered:

1) *Why is GSH in pancreas depleted during experimental acute pancreatitis ?*
2) *What is the relevance of the observed depletion of pancreatic GSH on pancreatitis ?*
3) *Does pharmacological increment of pancreatic GSH mitigate the damage due to acute pancreatitis ?*
4) *Is there any DNA oxidation in long term studies on experimental acute pancreatitis and in human AP, and if so, could this be a link to development of "post-pancreatitis" pancreatic cancer ?*
5) *Is there any evidence of ROS involvement in long term experimental acute pancreatitis ?*
6) *Is there any involvement of ROS in the multiple organ failure seen as a result of acute pancreatitis ?*

Further research is necessary in order to disclose these matters.

Summary (English)

The pathogenesis of acute pancreatitis (AP) is still little understood. It is generally accepted that an activation of pancreatic enzymes leads to "autodigestion" of the gland with local and/or remote organ failure as a result. As this common disease can have a high morbidity and lethality, much effort has been made to elucidate the initial events in order to discover a potential cure. Reactive oxygen species (ROS) that are produced in the organism can be harmful to cells if the capacity of the protective system, the antioxidants, is exceeded. In both experimental and human studies on AP there is evidence of an early involvement of ROS. Although the significance of this involvement is unclear, it has, nevertheless, been important to investigate it, as a potential pharmacological therapy is possible with the use of antioxidants.

In this study we wanted to examine the involvement of ROS in experimental AP. The study was conducted in two parts: Firstly, we wanted to characterize two models in rat; the taurocholate model (bile infusion into the pancreatobiliary duct) and the cerulein model (i.v. infusion of a cholecystokinin analogue). Secondly, we wanted to test our hypothesis: *Induction of AP would lead to an early depletion of the antioxidants ascorbic acid and glutathione, a simultaneous increase in their oxidized forms and an increase in markers of lipid peroxidation and DNA oxidation.* The methods used in the model characterizations were assessments of the following: Lipase and amylase activity in plasma, macroscopic variables such as peritoneal exudate and histological scoring. Both models were described with a time course study and additionally, the taurocholate model was described with a dose-response study. To test our hypothesis, the antioxidants and the markers of oxidative damage were measured in pancreatic tissue and in plasma over time.

As a result, we found both models were reproducible and resembled morphological and biochemical changes as seen in human AP. We found an early and moderate depletion of glutathione in both models and an increase in oxidized glutathione in the cerulein model. Ascorbic acid did not decrease nor did the oxidized form increase. Furthermore, no increase in markers of oxidative damage to the cells, was found. Conclusively, the study suggests no major involvement of ROS in the initial steps of these two experimental AP models.

Summary (Danish)

Patogenesen ved akut bugspytkirtelbetændelse, pancreatitis acuta (AP), er fortsat ukendt. En teori er, at der ved en aktivering af kirtlens fordøjelsesenzymerne, sker en "autofordøjelse" af organet med mulig skade på fjerntliggende organer. AP er en almindeligt forekommende sygdom med høj morbiditet og høj letalitet. En forståelse af mekanismerne ved den tidlige del af sygdommen er af stor interesse mhp. udviklingen af en effektiv behandling. Reaktive oksygen species (ROS) som til stadighed produceres i kroppen kan medføre celleskade, hvis den dannede mængde overstiger cellernes forsvarssystemer, antioxidanterne. Resultater fra både eksperimentelle og humane studier peger på, at ROS tidligt er involveret i AP. Betydningen af tilstedeværelsen af ROS ved AP er fortsat ikke afklaret, men åbner for potentielle farmakologiske behandlingsmuligheder med antioxidanter.

I denne afhandling har vi ønsket at undersøge forekomsten af ROS ved eksperimentel AP. Studiet blev udført i to dele: Først karakteriserede vi to rottemodeller. Den ene model var en taurocholat model (infusion af galde i den fælles udførsels gang for lever og pankreas), den anden var en cerulein model (i.v. infusion af en cholecystokinin analog). Dernæst testede vi hypotesen: *Induktion af AP vil medføre tidlig depletering af antioxidanterne ascorbinsyre og glutathion, en samtidig øgning af disse antioxidanters oksiderede former samt en øgning i markører for lipid peroxsidering og DNA oxidation.* Ved modelkarakteriseringen måltes: Lipase- og amylase aktiviteter i plasma, makroskopiske variable som fx. peritoneal eksudat samt histologisk scoring. Begge modeller blev beskrevet ved tidsstudier og taurocholat modellen yderligere ved et dosis-responsstudie. Ved hypotesetestningen måltes: Antioxidanter og markører for oxidativ celle skade i plasma og væv som følge af tid.

Vi fandt, at begge modeller var reproducerbare og lignede de morfologiske og biokemiske forandringer som ses ved human AP. Begge modeller havde en tidlig depletering af glutathion i pankreas og kun i ceruleinmodellen fandtes en stigning af oxideret glutathion. Vi fandt intet fald i ascorbinsyre og ingen stigning i dennes oxiderede form. Samtidig fandtes ingen af markørerne for oxidativ celleskade forhøjede. Vi konkluderer således, at ROS næppe bidrager væsentligt ved de tidlige stadier af eksperimentel AP i de to valgte modeller.

Abbreviations

AA	Ascorbic acid
AP	Acute pancreatitis
ATP	Adenosine triphosphate
Cat	Catalase
CCK	Cholecystokinin
CDE	Choline-deficient ethionine rich diet
CDL	Closed duodenal bop
dG	Deoxyguanosine
DHAA	Dehydroascorbic acid
DI	Duct infusion
DMSO	Dimethyl sulfoxide
DNA	Deoxyribonucleic acid
DOC	Duct occlusion model
DPTA	Diethylenetriamine-dipentacetic acid
DTNB	5,5'-dithiobis(2-nitrobenzoic acid)
EDTA	Ethylenediaminetetraacetic acid
ESR	Electron spin resonance
EXP	Ex-vivo perfusion
Gpx	Glutathione peroxidase
GSH	Glutathione
GSSG	Glutathione disulfide
H_2O_2	Hydrogen peroxide
HEPES	Hydroxyethyl piperazineethane
HPLC	High pressure liquid chromatography
ISC	Ischemia/reperfusion
MDA	Malondialdehyde
MPA	Metaphosphoric acid
NAC	N-acetyl cysteine
$^{\bullet}$OH	Hydroxyl radical
4-OH-TEMPO	4-hydroxy tetramethyl piperidinyloxy
8-oxodG	8-oxo-7,8-dihydro-2'-deoxoguanosine
PBD	Pancreatobiliary duct
PEG-SOD	Polyethylene glycol superoxide dismutase
PMN	Polymorphonuclear leukocyte
ROS	Reactive oxygen species
SEC	Secretagogue models
SOD	Superoxide dismutase

References

1. Worning H. Acute interstitial (edematous) pancreatitis in Denmark. In: Bradley III EL, editor. *Acute pancreatitis: Diagnosis and therapy.* New York: Raven Press, Ltd., 1994:265-9.

2. Wilson C, Imrie CW. Changing patterns of incidence and mortality from acute pancreatitis in Scotland, 1961-1985. *Br J Surg* 1990;**77**:731-4.

3. Jaakkola M, Nordback I. Pancreatitis in Finland between 1970 and 1989. *Gut* 1993;**34(9)**:1255-60.

4. Chiari H. Ueber selbstverdauung des menschlichen pankreas. *Zeitschrift für Heilkunde* 1896;**17**:69-96.

5. Opie EL. The etiology of acute hemorrhagic pancreatitis. *Johns Hopkins Hosp Bull* 1901;**12**:182-8.

6. Symmers WSC. Acute alcoholic pancreatitis. *Dublin Journal of Medical Science* 1917;**143**:244-7.

7. Fitz RH. Acute pancreatitis. A consideration of pancreatic hemmorrhage, hemorrhagic, suppurative, and gangrenous pancreatitis, and of disseminated fat-necrosis. *The Medical Journal* 1889;**35(8-10)**:197-204.

8. Kingsnorth A. Mediators in acute pancreatitis. *Scand J Gastroenterol Suppl* 1996;**31 Suppl. 219**:1-50.

9. Friess H, Weber A, Buchler M. Standards in monitoring acute experimental pancreatitis. [Review]. *Eur Surg Res* 1992;**24 Suppl 1**:1-13.

10. Halliwell B, Gutteridge JMC. Free radicals in biology and medicine. Claredon, Oxford: Oxford University Press, 1989.

11. Otamiri T, Sjodahl R. Oxygen radicals: their role in selected gastrointestinal disorders. [Review]. *Dig Dis* 1991;**9(3)**:133-41.

12. Sanfey H, Bulkley GB, Cameron JL. The role of oxygen-derived free radicals in the pathogenesis of acute pancreatitis. *Ann Surg* 1984;**200**:405-13.

13. Banerjee AK, Galloway SW, Kingsnorth AN. Experimental models of acute pancreatitis. [Review]. *Br J Surg* 1994;**81**:1096-103.

14. Aho HJ, Koskensalo SM, Nevalainen TJ. Experimental pancreatitis in the rat. Sodium taurocholate-induced acute haemorrhagic pancreatitis. *Scand J Gastroenterol* 1980;**15**:411-6.

15. Wedgwood KR, Farmer RC, Reber HA. A model of hemorrhagic pancreatitis in cats--role of 16,16-dimethyl prostaglandin E2. *Gastroenterology* 1986;**90**:32-9.

16. Senninger N, Moody FG, Coelho JC, Van Buren DH. The role of biliary obstruction in the pathogenesis of acute pancreatitis in the opossum. *Surgery* 1986;**99**:688-93.

17. Schmidt J, Rattner DW, Lewandrowski K, Compton CC, Mandavilli U, Knoefel WT, et al. A better model of acute pancreatitis for evaluating therapy. *Ann Surg* 1992;**215**:44-56.

18. Chetty U, Gilmour HM, Taylor TV. Experimental acute pancreatitis in the rat--a new model. *Gut* 1980;**21**:115-7.

19. Formela LJ, Wood LM, Whittaker M, Kingsnorth AN. Amelioration of experimental acute pancreatitis with a potent platelet-activating factor antagonist. *Br J Surg* 1994;**81**:1783-5.

20. Shibayama Y. Pancreatic venous stasis and endotoxaemia as aetiologic factors in acute haemorrhagic pancreatitis. *J Pathol* 1987;**152**:177-82.

21. Redha F, Uhlschmid G, Ammann RW, Freiburghaus AU. Injection of microspheres into pancreatic arteries causes acute hemorrhagic pancreatitis in the rat: a new animal model. *Pancreas* 1990;**5**:188-93.

22. Saharia P, Margolis S, Zuidema GD, Cameron JL. Acute pancreatitis with hyperlipemia: studies with an isolated perfused canine pancreas. *Surgery* 1977;**82**:60-7.

23. Lampel M, Kern HF. Acute interstitial pancreatitis in the rat induced by excessive doses of a pancreatic secretagogue. *Virchows Arch A Pathol Anat Histopathol* 1977;**373**:97-117.

24. Niederau C, Luthen R, Niederau MC, Grendell JH, Ferrell LD. Acute experimental hemorrhagic-necrotizing pancreatitis induced by feeding a choline-deficient, ethionine-supplemented diet. Methodology and standards. [Review]. *Eur Surg Res* 1992;**24 Suppl 1**:40-54.

25. De Almeida AL, Grossman MI. Experimental production of pancreatitis with ethionine. *Gastroenterology* 1952;**20**:554-77.

26. Thal A, Brackney E. Acute hemmorrhagic pancreatic necrosis produced by Schwartzman reaction. *JAMA* 1954;**155**:569-74.

27. Halliwell B. Free radicals, antioxidants, and human disease: curiosity, cause, or consequence?. [Review]. *Lancet* 1994;**344**:721-4.

28. Martinez-Cayuela M. Oxygen free radicals and human disease. [Review]. *Biochimie* 1995;**77**:147-61.

29. Jacob RA. The integrated antioxidant system. *Nutr Res (New York)* 1995;**15 (5)**:755-66.

30. Beckman JS, Beckman TW, Chen J, Marshall PA, Freeman BA. Apparent hydroxyl radical production by peroxynitrite: implications for endothelial injury from nitric oxide and superoxide. *Proc Natl Acad Sci U S A* 1990;**87**:1620-4.

31. Gutteridge JM. Lipid peroxidation and antioxidants as biomarkers of tissue damage. [Review]. *Clin Chem* 1995;**41(12 Pt 2)**:1819-28.

32. Meister A. Glutathione-ascorbic acid antioxidant system in animals. [Review]. *J Biol Chem* 1994;**269**:9397-400.

33. Frei B, England L, Ames BN. Ascorbate is an outstanding antioxidant in human blood plasma. *Proc Natl Acad Sci U S A* 1989;**86**:6377-81.

34. Meister A. On the antioxidant effects of ascorbic acid and glutathione. [Review]. *Biochem Pharmacol* 1992;**44**:1905-15.

35. Luthen RE, Grendell JH. Thiol metabolism and acute pancreatitis: trying to make the pieces fit [editorial]. *Gastroenterology* 1994;**107**:888-92.

36. Hwang C, Sinskey AJ, Lodish HF. Oxidized redox state of glutathione in the endoplasmic reticulum. *Science* 1992;**257**:1496-502.

37. Scheele G, Jacoby R. Conformational changes associated with proteolytic processing of presecretory proteins allow glutathione-catalyzed formation of native disulfide bonds. *J Biol Chem* 1982;**257**:12277-82.

38. Jewell SA, Bellomo G, Thor H, Orrenius S, Smith M. Bleb formation in hepatocytes during drug metabolism is caused by disturbances in thiol and calcium ion homeostasis. *Science* 1982;**217**:1257-9.

39. Stenson WF, Lobos E, Wedner HJ. Glutathione depletion inhibits amylase release in guinea pig pancreatic acini. *Am J Physiol* 1983;**244**:G273-7.

40. Saluja A, Rutherford L, Nishino H, Runzi M, Saluja M, Cui ZJ, et al. Depletion of pancreatic glutathione results in the inhibition of secretagogue-stimulated amylase secretion but does not prevent secretagogue-induced rise in intracellular calcium in rat acini. *Gastroenterology* 1994;**106(4)**:A320.

41.   Githens S. Glutathione metabolism in the pancreas compared with that in the liver, kidney, and small intestine. [Review]. *Int J Pancreatol* 1991;**8**:97-109.

42.   Jain A, Martensson J, Mehta T, Krauss AN, Auld PA, Meister A. Ascorbic acid prevents oxidative stress in glutathione-deficient mice: effects on lung type 2 cell lamellar bodies, lung surfactant, and skeletal muscle. *Proc Natl Acad Sci U S A* 1992;**89**:5093-7.

43.   Martensson J, Meister A, Martensson J. Glutathione deficiency decreases tissue ascorbate levels in newborn rats: ascorbate spares glutathione and protects. *Proc Natl Acad Sci U S A* 1991;**88**:4656-60.

44.   Sies H, Stahl W. Vitamins E and C, beta-carotene, and other carotenoids as antioxidants. [Review]. *Am J Clin Nutr* 1995;**62**:1315S-21S.

45.   Niki E. Action of ascorbic acid as a scavenger of active and stable oxygen radicals. *Am J Clin Nutr* 1991;**54**:1119S-24S.

46.   Rose RC, Bode AM. Analysis of water-soluble antioxidants by high-pressure liquid chromatography. *Biochem J* 1995;**306 (Pt 1)**:101-5.

47.   Zhou A, Thorn NA. High ascorbic acid content in the rat endocrine pancreas. *Diabetologia* 1991;**34(11)**:839-42.

48.   Frei B, Stocker R, Ames BN. Antioxidant defenses and lipid peroxidation in human blood plasma. *Proc Natl Acad Sci U S A* 1988;**85**:9748-52.

49.   Frei B, Stocker R, England L, Ames BN. Ascorbate: the most effective antioxidant in human blood plasma. *Advances in Experimental Medicine & Biology* 1990;**264**:155-63.

50.   Niki E, Noguchi N, Tsuchihashi H, Gotoh N. Interaction among vitamin C, vitamin E, and beta-carotene. *Am J Clin Nutr* 1995;**62(6 Suppl)**:1322S-6S.

51.   Esterbauer H, Schaur RJ, Zollner H. Chemistry and biochemistry of 4-hydroxynonenal, malonaldehyde and related aldehydes. [Review]. *Free Radical Biology & Medicine* 1991;**11(1)**:81-128.

52.   Loft S, Poulsen HE. Cancer risk and oxidative DNA damage in man. *J Mol Med* 1996;**74**:297-312.

53.   Schoenberg MH, Buchler M, Helfen M, Beger HG. Role of oxygen radicals in experimental acute pancreatitis. [Review]. *Eur Surg Res* 1992;**24 Suppl 1**:74-84.

54.   Littauer A, de Groot H. Release of reactive oxygen by hepatocytes on reoxygenation: three phases and role of mitochondria. *Am J Physiol* 1992;**262**:G1015-20.

55.   Saluja A, Hashimoto S, Saluja M, Powers RE, Meldolesi J, Steer ML. Subcellular redistribution of lysosomal enzymes during caerulein-induced pancreatitis. *Am J Physiol* 1987;**253**:G508-16.

56.   Manabe T, Hirano T, Ando K, Yotsumoto F, Tobe T. Effect of prostaglandin E2 on cellular, lysosomal and mitochondrial fragility in caerulein-induced pancreatitis in rats. *Hepatogastroenterology* 1993;**40**:463-6.

57.   Smith JA. Neutrophils, host defense, and inflammation: a double-edged sword. [Review]. *J Leukoc Biol* 1994;**56**:672-86.

58.   Silverman M, Ilardi C, Bank S, Kranz V, Lendvai S. Effects of the cholecystokinin receptor antagonist L-364,718 on experimental pancreatitis in mice. *Gastroenterology* 1989;**96**:186-92.

59.   Gilrane TB, Glover WJ, Granger DN, Holt SL, Powers RE. A temporal role of neutrophils in the pathogenesis of caerulein -induced acute pancreatitis. *Pancreas* 1989;**4 (5)**:617.

60.   Guice KS, Oldham KT, Johnson KJ, Kunkel RG, Morganroth ML, Ward PA. Pancreatitis-induced acute lung injury. An ARDS model. *Ann Surg* 1988;**208**:71-7.

61. Willemer S, Feddersen CO, Karges W, Adler G. Lung injury in acute experimental pancreatitis in rats. I. Morphological studies. *Int J Pancreatol* 1991;**8**:305-21.

62. Gross V, Leser HG, Heinisch A, Scholmerich J. Inflammatory mediators and cytokines--new aspects of the pathophysiology and assessment of severity of acute pancreatitis?. [Review]. *Hepatogastroenterology* 1993;**40**:522-30.

63. Murakami H, Nakao A, Kishimoto W, Nakano M, Takagi H. Detection of O2-generation and neutrophil accumulation in rat lungs after acute necrotizing pancreatitis. *Surgery* 1995;**118**:547-54.

64. Bulkley GB. Reactive oxygen metabolites and reperfusion injury: aberrant triggering of reticuloendothelial function. [Review]. *Lancet* 1994;**344**:934-6.

65. Schoenberg MH, Buchler M, Beger HG. Oxygen radicals in experimental acute pancreatitis. [Review]. *Hepatogastroenterology* 1994;**41**:313-9.

66. Sanfey H, Bulkley GB, Cameron JL. The pathogenesis of acute pancreatitis. The source and role of oxygen-derived free radicals in three different experimental models. *Ann Surg* 1985;**201**:633-9.

67. Sarr MG, Bulkley GB, Cameron JL. Temporal efficacy of allopurinol during the induction of pancreatitis in the ex vivo perfused canine pancreas. *Surgery* 1987;**101**:342-6.

68. Nonaka A, Manabe T, Asano N, Kyogoku T, Imanishi K, Tamura K, et al. Direct ESR measurement of free radicals in mouse pancreatic lesions. *Int J Pancreatol* 1989;**5**:203-11.

69. Gough DB, Boyle B, Joyce WP, Delaney CP, McGeeney KF, Gorey TF, et al. Free radical inhibition and serial chemiluminescence in evolving experimental pancreatitis. *Br J Surg* 1990;**77**:1256-9.

70. Kishimoto W, Nakao A, Nakano M, Takahashi A, Inaba H, Takagi H. Detection of superoxide free radicals in rats with acute pancreatitis. *Pancreas* 1995;**11**:122-6.

71. Peralta J, Reides C, Garcia S, Llesuy S, Pargament G, Carreras MC, et al. Oxidative stress in rodent closed duodenal loop pancreatitis. *Int J Pancreatol* 1996;**19**:61-9.

72. Nordback IH, Olson JL, Chacko VP, Cameron JL. Detailed characterization of experimental acute alcoholic pancreatitis. *Surgery* 1995;**117**:41-9.

73. Guice KS, Miller DE, Oldham KT, Townsend Jr CM, Thompson JC. Superoxide dismutase and catalase: a possible role in established pancreatitis. *Am J Surg* 1986;**151**:163-9.

74. Wisner J, Green D, Ferrell L, Renner I. Evidence for a role of oxygen derived free radicals in the pathogenesis of caerulein induced acute pancreatitis in rats. *Gut* 1988;**29**:1516-23.

75. Schoenberg MH, Buchler M, Gaspar M, Stinner A, Younes M, Melzner I, et al. Oxygen free radicals in acute pancreatitis of the rat. *Gut* 1990;**31**:1138-43.

76. Wisner JR, Renner IG. Allopurinol attenuates caerulein induced acute pancreatitis in the rat. *Gut* 1988;**29**:926-9.

77. Sledzinski Z, Wozniak M, Antosiewicz J, Lezoche E, Familiari M, Bertoli E, et al. Protective effect of 4-hydroxy-TEMPO, a low molecular weight superoxide dismutase mimic, on free radical toxicity in experimental pancreatitis. *Int J Pancreatol* 1995;**18**:153-60.

78. Nonaka A, Manabe T, Kyogoku T, Tamura K, Tobe T. Evidence for a role of free radicals by synthesized scavenger, 2-octadecylascorbic acid, in cerulein-induced mouse acute pancreatitis. *Dig Dis Sci* 1992;**37**:274-9.

79. Steer ML, Rutledge PL, Powers RE, Saluja M, Saluja AK. The role of oxygen-derived free radicals in two models of experimental acute pancreatitis: effects of catalase,

superoxide dismutase, dimethylsulfoxide, and allopurinol. *Klin Wochenschr* 1991;**69**:1012-7.

80. Niederau C, Niederau M, Borchard F, Ude K, Luthen R, Strohmeyer G, et al. Effects of antioxidants and free radical scavengers in three different models of acute pancreatitis. *Pancreas* 1992;**7**:486-96.

81. Schoenberg MH, Buchler M, Baczako K, Bultmann B, Younes M, Gasper M, et al. The involvement of oxygen radicals in acute pancreatitis. *Klin Wochenschr* 1991;**69**:1025-31.

82. Closa D, Bulbena O, Rosello-Catafau J, Fernandez-Cruz L, Gelpi E. Effect of prostaglandins and superoxide dismutase administration on oxygen free radical production in experimental acute pancreatitis. *Inflammation* 1993;**17**:563-71.

83. Wang XD, Deng XM, Haraldsen P, Andersson R, Ihse I. Antioxidant and calcium channel blockers counteract endothelial barrier injury induced by acute pancreatitis in rats. *Scand J Gastroenterol* 1995;**30**:1129-36.

84. Blind PJ, Marklund SL, Stenling R, Dahlgren ST. Parenteral superoxide dismutase plus catalase diminishes pancreatic edema in sodium taurocholate-induced pancreatitis in the rat. *Pancreas* 1988;**3**:563-7.

85. Lankisch PG, Pohl U, Otto J, Wereszczynska-Siemiatkowska U, Grone HJ. Xanthine oxidase inhibitor in acute experimental pancreatitis in rats and mice. *Pancreas* 1989;**4**:436-40.

86. Rutledge PL, Saluja AK, Powers RE, Steer ML. Role of oxygen-derived free radicals in diet-induced hemorrhagic pancreatitis in mice. *Gastroenterology* 1987;**93**:41-7.

87. Nonaka A, Manabe T, Tobe T. Effect of a new synthetic ascorbic acid derivative as a free radical scavenger on the development of acute pancreatitis in mice. *Gut* 1991;**32**:528-32.

88. Hirano T, Furuyama H, Kawakami Y, Ando K, Tsuchitani T. Protective effects of prophylaxis with a protease inhibitor and a free radical scavenger against a temporary ischemia model of pancreatitis. *Can J Surg* 1995;**38**:241-8.

89. Koiwai T, Oguchi H, Kawa S, Yanagisawa Y, Kobayashi T, Homma T. The role of oxygen free radicals in experimental acute pancreatitis in the rat. *Int J Pancreatol* 1989;**5**:135-43.

90. Tsimoyiannis EC, Tsimoyiannis JC, Lekkas ET, Betzios JP, Pange P, Kotoulas OB. Role of oxygen radicals in experimental acute pancreatitis induced by closed duodenal loop. *Hellenic Journal of Gastroenterology* 1993;**6(1)**:27-34.

91. Luthen RE, Niederau C, Grendell JH. Glutathione and ATP levels, subcellular distribution of enzymes, and permeability of duct system in rabbit pancreas following intravenous administration of alcohol and cerulein. *Dig Dis Sci* 1994;**39**:871-9.

92. Dabrowski A, Gabryelewicz A, Wereszczynska-Siemiatkowska U, Chyczewski L. Oxygen-derived free radicals in cerulein-induced acute pancreatitis. *Scand J Gastroenterol* 1988;**23**:1245-9.

93. Dabrowski A, Chwiecko M. Oxygen radicals mediate depletion of pancreatic sulfhydryl compounds in rats with cerulein-induced acute pancreatitis. *Digestion* 1990;**47**:15-9.

94. Luthen R, Niederau C, Grendell JH. Intrapancreatic zymogen activation and levels of ATP and glutathione during caerulein pancreatitis in rats. *Am J Physiol* 1995;**268**:G592-604.

95. Nonaka A, Manabe T, Kyogoku T, Tamura K, Tobe T. Changes in lipid peroxide and oxygen radical scavengers in cerulein-induced acute pancreatitis. Imbalance between the offense and defense systems. *Digestion* 1990;**47**:130-7.

96. Neuschwander-Tetri BA, Ferrell LD, Sukhabote RJ, Grendell JH. Glutathione monoethyl ester ameliorates caerulein-induced pancreatitis in the mouse. *J Clin Invest* 1992;**89**:109-16.

97. Schoenberg MH, Buchler M, Younes M, Kirchmayr R, Bruckner UB, Beger HG. Effect of antioxidant treatment in rats with acute hemorrhagic pancreatitis. *Dig Dis Sci* 1994;**39**:1034-40.

98. Dabrowski A, Gabryelewicz A. Oxidative stress. An early phenomenon characteristic of acute experimental pancreatitis. *Int J Pancreatol* 1992;**12**:193-9.

99. Nonaka A, Manabe T, Tamura K, Asano N, Imanishi K, Tobe T. Changes of xanthine oxidase, lipid peroxide and superoxide dismutase in mouse acute pancreatitis. *Digestion* 1989;**43**:41-6.

100. Schoenberg MH, Buchler M, Pietrzyk C, Uhl W, Birk D, Eisele S, et al. Lipid peroxidation and glutathione metabolism in chronic pancreatitis. *Pancreas* 1995;**10**:36-43.

101. Lu FJ, Lin JT, Wang HP, Huang WC. A simple, sensitive, non-stimulated photon counting system for detection of superoxide anion in whole blood. *Experientia* 1996;**52**:141-4.

102. Braganza JM, Scott P, Bilton D, Schofield D, Chaloner C, Shiel N, et al. Evidence for early oxidative stress in acute pancreatitis. Clues for correction. *Int J Pancreatol* 1995;**17(1)**:69-81.

103. Waele BD, Vierendeels T, Willems G. Vitamin status in patients with acute pancreatitis. *Clin Nutr* 1992;**11**:83-6.

104. Scott P, Bruce C, Schofield D, Shiel N, Braganza JM, McCloy RF. Vitamin C status in patients with acute pancreatitis. *Br J Surg* 1993;**80**:750-4.

105. Guyan PM, Uden S, Braganza JM. Heightened free radical activity in pancreatitis. *Free Radic Biol Med* 1990;**8**:347-54.

106. Honjo K, Uehara S, Hirano F, Furukawa S, Hirayama A. Changes of lipid peroxides and their scavengers in patients with acute and chronic pancreatitis. In: Hayaishi O, Niki E, Kondo M, Yoshikawa T, editors. *Medical, biochemical and chemical aspects of free radicals.* Amsterdam: Elsevier, 1988:1025-8.

107. Kuklinski B, Buchner M, Schweder R, Nagel R. [Acute pancreatitis--a free radical disease. Decrease in fatality with sodium selenite (Na2SeO3) therapy]. *Z Gesamte Inn Med* 1991;**46**:145-9.

108. Schofield D, Summan M, Shiel N, Sharer NM, Braganza JM. Blood glutathione and adenylates in acute pancreatitis. *Biochem Soc Trans* 1993;**21**:450S.

109. Buchler M, Friess H, Uhl W, Beger HG. Clinical relevance of experimental acute pancreatitis. [Review]. *Eur Surg Res* 1992;**24 Suppl 1**:85-8.

110. Adler G, Rohr G, Kern HF. Alteration of membrane fusion as a cause of acute pancreatitis in the rat. *Dig Dis Sci* 1982;**27**:993-1002.

111. Wereszczynska-Siemiatkowska U, Nebendahl K, Pohl U, Otto J, Groene HJ, Wilms H, et al. Influence of buprenorphine on acute experimental pancreatitis. *Res Exp Med (Berl)* 1987;**187**:211-6.

112. Wang XD, Andersson R, Kruse P, Ihse I. Carbon dioxide transport in rats with acute pancreatitis. *International J Pancreatol* 1996;**19(2)**:103-12.

113. Bieger W, Martin-Achard A, Bassler M, Kern HF. Studies on intracellular transport of secretory proteins in the rat exocrine pancreas. IV. Stimulation by in vivo infusion of caerulein. *Cell & Tissue Research* 1976;**165**:435-53.

114. Ziegenhorn J, Neumann U, Knitsch KW, Zwez W. Determination of serum lipase. *Clin Chem* 1979;**25 (6)**:103-13.

114b Kruse-Jarres, JD, Kaiser, C. Evaluation of a new α-amylase assay using 4.6-ethylidene-(G7)-1-4-nitrophenyl-(G1)- α-D-maltoheptaoside as substrate. J Clin Chem Clin Biochem 1989;27:103-13.

115. Spormann H, Sokolowski A, Letko G. Effect of temporary ischemia upon development and histological patterns of acute pancreatitis in the rat. *Pathol Res Pract* 1989;**184**:507-13.

116. Tani S, Otsuki M, Itoh H, Fujii M, Nakamura T, Oka T, et al. Histologic and biochemical alterations in experimental acute pancreatitis induced by supramaximal caerulein stimulation. *Int J Pancreatol* 1987;**2**:337-48.

117. Siegel S, Castellan NJ. Non parametric statistics for the behavioral sciences. New York: McGraw-Hill, 1988.

118. Anderson ME. Enzymatic and chemical methods for the determination of glutathione. In: Dolphin D, Poulson R, Avramovic O, editors. *Coenzymes and cofactors: Glutathione.* New York: John Wiley, 1989:339-66.

119. Lykkesfeldt J, Loft S, Poulsen HE. Determination of ascorbic acid and dehydroascorbic acid in plasma by high-performance liquid chromatography with coulometric detection--are they reliable biomarkers of oxidative stress?. *Anal Biochem* 1995;**229**:329-35.

120. Fischer-Nielsen A, Corcoran GB, Poulsen HE, Kamendulis LM, Loft S. Menadione-induced DNA fragmentation without 8-oxo-2'-deoxyguanosine formation in isolated rat hepatocytes. *Biochem Pharmacol* 1995;**49(10)**:1469-74.

121. Lowry OH, Rosebrough NJ, Farr AL, Randall RF. Protein measurement with the Folin phenol reagent. *J Biol Chem* 1951;**193**:265-75.

122. Lankisch PG, Ihse I. Bile-induced acute experimental pancreatitis. *Scand J Gastroenterol* 1987;**22**:257-60.

123. Armstrong CP, Taylor TV, Torrance HB. Pressure, volume and the pancreas. *Gut* 1985;**26**:615-24.

124. Aho HJ, Suonpaa K, Ahola RA, Nevalainen TJ. Experimental pancreatitis in the rat. Ductal factors in sodium taurocholate-induced acute pancreatitis. *Exp Pathol* 1984;**25**:73-9.

125. Hansson K. Experimental and clinical studies in aetiologic role of bile reflux in acute pancreatitis. *Acta Chir Scand Suppl* 1967;**375**:102.

126. Foulis AK. Pathology of acute pancreatitis. In: Glazer G, Ranson JHC, editors. *Acute pancreatitis. Experimental and clinical aspects of pathogenesis and management.* London: Baillière Tindall, 1988:194-206.

127. Wanke M. Experimental acute pancreatitis. [Review]. *Curr Top Pathol* 1970;**52**:64-142.

128. Maringhini A, Ciambra M, Patti R, Randazzo MA, Dardanoni G, Mancuso L, et al. Ascites, pleural, and pericardial effusions in acute pancreatitis. A prospective study of incidence, natural history, and prognostic role. *Digestive Diseases & Sciences* 1996;**41**:848-52.

129. Courtois P, Art G, Vertongen F, Franckson JR. Evolution of serum amylase, lipase and immunoreactive trypsin during pancreatitis attacks. *Ann Biol Clin (Paris)* 1985;**43**:127-31.

130. Papp M, Varga G, Folly G, Törcsvári V. The fate of pancreatic secretory proteins in the blood circulation of dogs and rats. *Acta Physiol Acad Sci Hung* 1982;**59 (4)**:329-39.

131. Aho HJ, Nevalainen TJ, Aho AJ. Experimental pancreatitis in the rat. Development of pancreatic necrosis, ischemia and edema after intraductal sodium taurocholate injection. *Eur Surg Res* 1983;**15**:28-36.

132. Schmidt J, Lewandrowski K, Fernandez-del Castillo C, Mandavilli U, Compton CC, Warshaw AL, et al. Histopathologic correlates of serum amylase activity in acute experimental pancreatitis. *Dig Dis Sci* 1992;**37**:1426-33.

133. Gullick HD. Relation of the magnitude of blood enzyme elevation to severity of exocrine pancreatic disease. *Am J Dig Dis* 1973;**18**:375-83.

134. Lankisch PG, Koop H, Winckler K, Kunze H, Vogt W. Indomethacin treatment of acute experimental pancreatitis in the rat. *Scand J Gastroenterol* 1978;**13**:629-33.

135. Closa D, Hotter G, Prats N, Bulbena O, Rosello-Catafau J, Fernandez-Cruz L, et al. Prostanoid generation in early stages of acute pancreatitis: a role for nitric oxide. *Inflammation* 1994;**18**:469-80.

136. Samuel I, Toriumi Y, Wilcockson DP, Turkelson CM, Solomon TE, Joehl RJ. Bile and pancreatic juice replacement ameliorates early ligation-induced acute pancreatitis in rats. *Am J Surg* 1995;**169**:391-9.

137. Opie EL. The relation of cholelithiasis to disease of the pancreas and to fat necrosis. *John Hopkins Hosp Bull* 1901;**12**:19-21.

138. McCutcheon AD. Reflux of duodenal contents in the pathogenesis of pancreatitis. *Gut* 1964;**5**:260-5.

139. Carr-Locke DL, Gregg JA. Endoscopic manometry of pancreatic and biliary sphincter zones in man. Basal results in healthy volunteers. *Digestive Diseases & Sciences* 1981;**26(1)**:7-15.

140. Whitrock RM, Hine D, Crane J, McCorkel HJ. The effect of bile flow through the pancreas. *Dig Dis Sci* 1955;**38**:122-33.

141. Saluja AK, Saluja M, Printz H, Zavertnik A, Sengupta A, Steer ML. Experimental pancreatitis is mediated by low-affinity cholecystokinin receptors that inhibit digestive enzyme secretion. *Proc Natl Acad Sci U S A* 1989;**86**:8968-71.

142. Kern HF, Adler G, Scheele GA. Structural and biochemical characterization of maximal and supramaximal hormonal stimulation of rat exocrine pancreas. *Scand J Gastroenterol Suppl* 1985;**112**:20-9.

143. Watanabe O, Baccino FM, Steer ML, Meldolesi J. Supramaximal caerulein stimulation and ultrastructure of rat pancreatic acinar cell: early morphological changes during development of experimental pancreatitis. *Am J Physiol* 1984;**246**:G457-67.

144. Gorelick FS, Adler G, Kern HF. Cerulein-induced pancreatitis. In: Go W, editor. *The pancreas: Biology, pathobiology and diseases.* New York: Raven Press, 1993:501-26.

145. Elsasser HP, Adler G, Kern HF. Fibroblast structure and function during regeneration from hormone-induced acute pancreatitis in the rat. *Pancreas* 1989;**4**:169-78.

146. Schmidt J, Compton CC, Rattner DW, Lewandrowski K, Warshaw AL. Late histopathologic changes and healing in an improved rodent model of acute necrotizing pancreatitis. *Digestion* 1995;**56**:246-52.

147. Furukawa M, Kimura T, Sumii T, Yamaguchi H, Nawata H. Role of local pancreatic blood flow in development of hemorrhagic pancreatitis induced by stress in rats. *Pancreas* 1993;**8**:499-505.

148. Adler G, Kern HF. Fine structural and biochemical studies in human acute pancreatitis. In: Gyr KE, Singer MV, Sarles H, editors. *Pancreatitis - Concepts and classification.* Amsterdam: Elsevier Science Publishers B.V., 1984:37-42.

149. Willemer S, Adler G. Histochemical and ultrastructural characteristics of tubular complexes in human acute pancreatitis. *Dig Dis Sci* 1989;**34**:46-55.

150. Marsh WH, Vukov GA, Conradi EC. Acute pancreatitis after cutaneous exposure to an organophosphate insecticide. *Am J Gastroenterol* 1988;**83**:1158-60.

151. Bartholomew C. Acute scorpion pancreatitis in Trinidad. *Br Med J* 1970;**1**:666-8.

152. Dressel TD, Goodale Jr RL, Arneson MA, Borner JW. Pancreatitis as a complication of anticholinesterase insecticide intoxication. *Ann Surg* 1979;**189**:199-204.

153. Gronroos JM, Aho HJ, Nevalainen TJ. Cholinergic hypothesis of alcoholic pancreatitis. [Review]. *Dig Dis* 1992;**10**:38-45.

154. Willemer S, Kloppel G, Kern HF, Adler G. Immunocytochemical and morphometric analysis of acinar zymogen granules in human acute pancreatitis. *Virchows Arch A Pathol Anat Histopathol* 1989;**415**:115-23.

155. Willemer S, Elsasser HP, Adler G. Hormone-induced pancreatitis. [Review]. *Eur Surg Res* 1992;**24 Suppl 1**:29-39.

156. Halliwell B. Mechanisms involved in the generation of free radicals. *Pathol Biol (Paris)* 1996;**44 (1)**:6-13.

157. Janzen EG, Poyer JL, Schaefer CF, Downs PE, DuBose CM. Biological spin trapping. II. Toxicity of nitrone spin traps: dose-ranging in the rat. *Journal of Biochemical & Biophysical Methods* 1995;**30(4)**:239-47.

158. Neuschwander-Tetri BA, Barnidge M, Janney CG. Cerulein-induced pancreatic cysteine depletion: prevention does not diminish acute pancreatitis in the mouse. *Gastroenterology* 1994;**107**:824-30.

159. Martensson J, Meister A. Glutathione deficiency increases hepatic ascorbic acid synthesis in adult mice. *Proc Natl Acad Sci U S A* 1992;**89**:11566-8.

160. Maellaro E, Casini AF, Del Bello B, Comporti M. Lipid peroxidation and antioxidant systems in the liver injury produced by glutathione depleting agents. *Biochem Pharmacol* 1990;**39**:1513-21.

161. Martensson J, Jain A, Meister A. Glutathione is required for intestinal function. *Proc Natl Acad Sci U S A* 1990;**87**:1715-9.

162. Coursin DB, Cihla HP. The pulmonary effects of buthionine sulfoximine treatment and glutathione depletion in rats. *Am Rev Respir Dis* 1988;**138(6)**:1471-9.

163. Tu B, Wallin A, Moldeus P, Cotgreave I. The cytoprotective roles of ascorbate and glutathione against nitrogen dioxide toxicity in human endothelial cells. *Toxicology* 1995;**98(1-3)**:125-36.

164. Horton JW, Walker PB. Oxygen radicals, lipid peroxidation, and permeability changes after intestinal ischemia and reperfusion. *J Appl Physiol* 1993;**74(4)**:1515-20.

165. Loft S, Larsen PN, Rasmussen A, Fischer-Nielsen A, Bondesen S, Kirkegaard P, et al. Oxidative DNA damage after transplantation of the liver and small intestine in pigs. *Transplantation* 1995;**59(1)**:16-20.

166. Sai K, Takagi A, Umemura T, Hasegawa R, Kurokawa Y. Relation of 8-hydroxydeoxyguanosine formation in rat kidney to lipid peroxidation, glutathione level and relative organ weight after a single administration of potassium bromate. *Jpn J Cancer Res* 1991;**82(2)**:165-9.

167. Sai K, Umemura T, Takagi A, Hasegawa R, Kurokawa Y. The protective role of glutathione, cysteine and vitamin C against oxidative DNA damage induced in rat kidney by potassium bromate. *Jpn J Cancer Res* 1992;**83(1)**:45-51.

168. Park JW, Floyd RA. Lipid peroxidation products mediate the formation of 8-hydroxydeoxyguanosine in DNA. *Free Radical Biology & Medicine* 1992;**12(4)**:245-50.

169. Bansal P, Sonnenberg A. Pancreatitis is a risk factor for pancreatic cancer. *Gastroenterology* 1995;**109(1)**:247-51.

170. Ekbom A, McLaughlin JK, Karlsson BM, Nyren O, Gridley G, Adami HO, et al. Pancreatitis and pancreatic cancer: a population-based study. *J Natl Cancer Inst* 1994;**86**:625-7.

171. Tran DD, Cuesta MA, Schneider AJ, Wesdorp RI. Prevalence and prediction of multiple organ system failure and mortality in acute pancreatitis. *J Crit Care* 1993;**8**:145-53.

172. Del Maestro RF. An approach to free radicals in medicine and biology. *Acta Physiol Scand* 1980;**Supplementum. 49**:153-68.

Appendix

Technical features for the pressure controlled infusion pump

Lab-Vision
Infusion Pump
Model IP-0150

Type 0, December 1995

Features:

* Menu driven
* Accept plastic syringes
* Microprocessor motor control
* Alphanumeric LCD

The pump is configured via the three front panel keys. Settings can even be changed while the pump is running.

Nonvolatile memory stores and retains settings even when the pump is turned off.

System Components:

* Infusion pump controller
* Actuator unit
* Baxter Uniflow disposable pressure transducer model 43-600
* Transducer connection cable
* 230VAC power cord

Specifications:

Range   : 1 - 50 cm H_2O
Syringe size   : 1.0 ml
Max flow   : ~0.2 ml/min

Transducer data   according to Baxter   spec.:
Linearity   : ± 1% or ± 1 mm Hg
Zero offset   : < ± 40 mm Hg
Zero thermal drift :   ± 0.3 mm Hg/ °C

System linearity   : <   ± 1 cmH_2O*

* See linearity test sheet.

Error messages:

Error 1: Actuator missing.
- The actuator unit is not properly connected, check the cable and plug.

Error 2: Time out.
- The pressure was below the lower limit for too long. Flow rate is appr. 0.2 ml/min for 15 sec. when pressure is below lower limit. An empty syringe or faulty tube connection might be the reason. The pump is stopped. If the problem persist, decrement the lower limit.

Error 3: P > SETP+5 cmH2O
- The measured pressure exceeded the upper limit pressure by 5 cmH2O. The pump is stopped.

Operating instructions:

Setting up the pump is a straight forward process. Plug the power cord in to an earthen power source. Connect the actuator unit and the transducer to the controller via the transducer cable. Switch on the power switch at the rear of the controller. Allow 15 min. of warm up time.

On start-up, the display toggles between three product information lines, indicating a correct start. Hit any key to enter Stand By mode.

In Stand By mode, the two user defined limits are shown.

Pressing ^ and v simultaneously enters the Setup mode. If the pump is not running, the Calibration mode is entered. This mode allows for zero adjusting the transducer (against air). Use a small screw driver to turn the CAL adjustment screw on the front panel until a pressure reading of   0.0 cm H_2O is reached.

Hit the RUN/STOP key to jump to next Setup item which is used to edit the lower limit. Use ^ and v to increment/decrement the value. Minimum is 1 cmH$_2$O and maximum is upper limit - 5 cm H_2O.

To edit the upper limit, hit the RUN/STOP key. Minimum for the upper limit is lower limit +
5 cm H_2O and maximum is 50 cm H_2O.

Press the RUN/STOP key to exit Setup mode and return to either Stand By or Run mode, dependent on which one was selected at the time Setup mode was chosen.

In Stand By mode, the RUN/STOP key starts and stops the pump. This key is also used to recover from any error condition encountered during a run.

The pump is reset by the power switch.

NOTE 1: User must manually stop the pump when syringe is empty, in order to avoid damage of the actuator unit.

NOTE 2: It is crucial that the tubing system is absolutely free from air bubbles, otherwise unpredictable behaviour of the pressure regulaton will occur.

IMPORTANT: Designs and specifications are subject to change without notice.   The user is totally responsible for correct use and performance of this product and in no event shall **Lab-Vision** be liable for incidental or indirect damages of any kind arising from the use of this product.

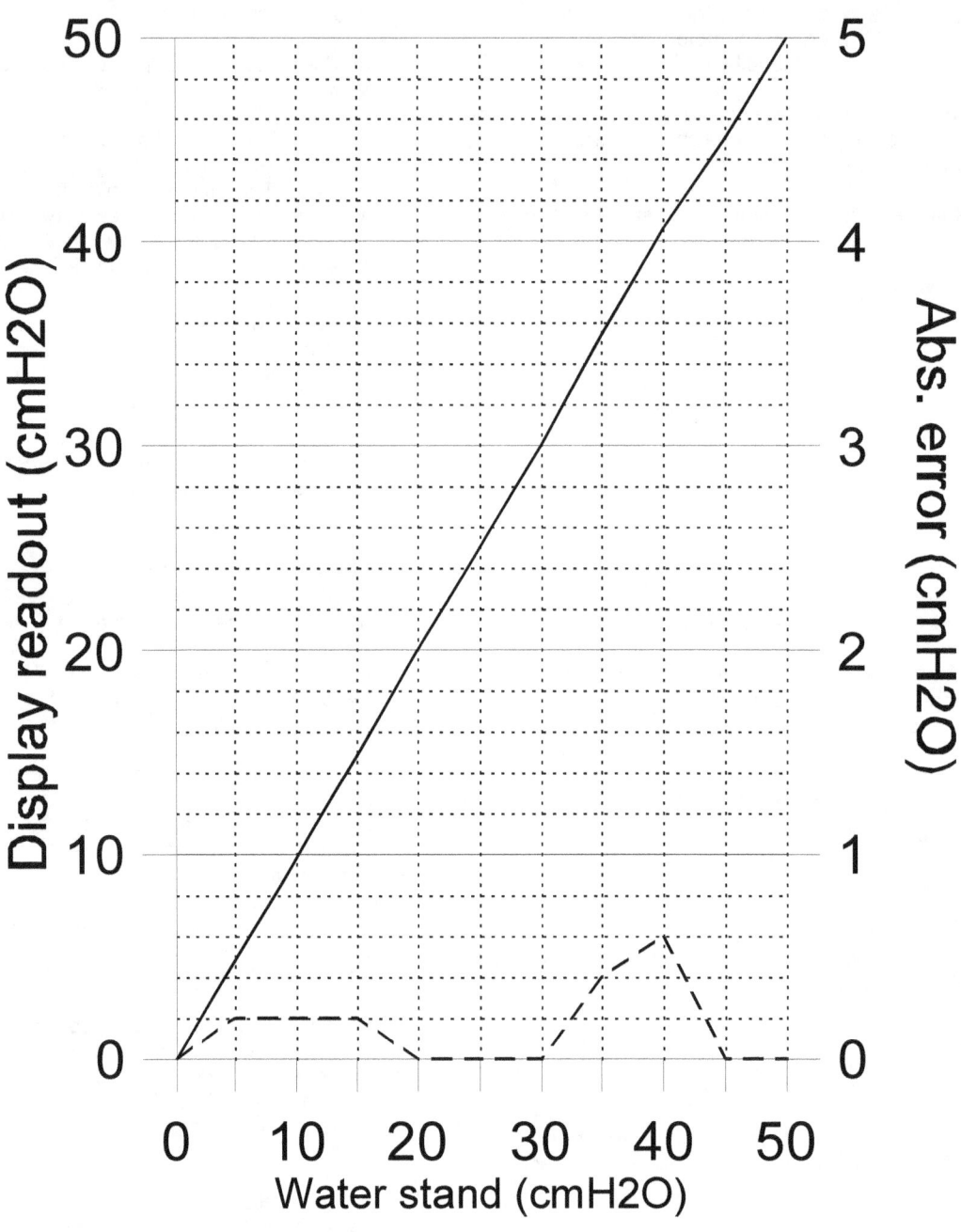

Lab-Vision IP-0150   Date: 13.12.

Linearity test. Amp. cal. at 50 cmH2O.

- - - - - - Absolute error (Y2)

Light microscopic pictures of the pancreas from the taurocholate time course study

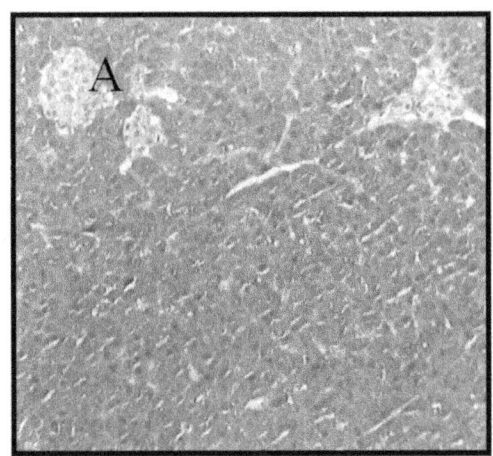

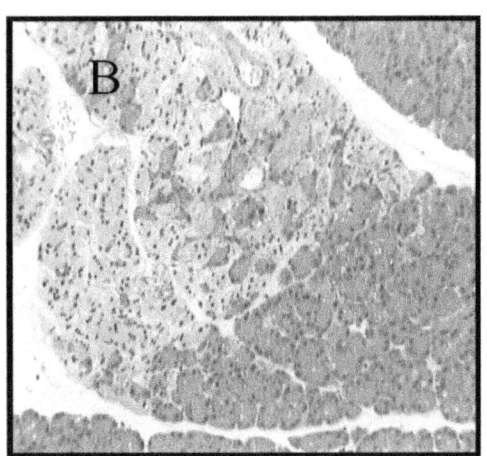

A: Normal pancreas from control rat (H.E. x 100)

B: 3 hours after 3% sodium taurocholate injection into PBD with the histo-pathological changes: Interstitial edema, acinar cell necrosis (focal and sublobular) (H.E. x 100)

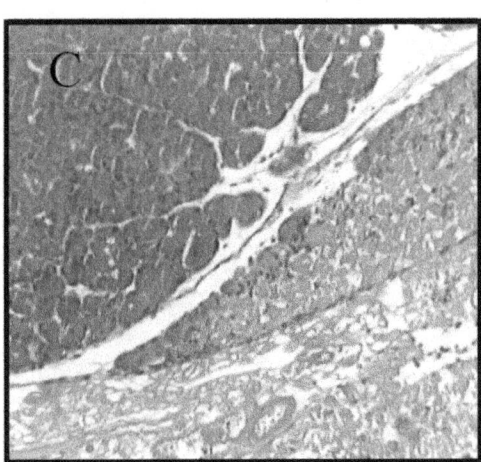

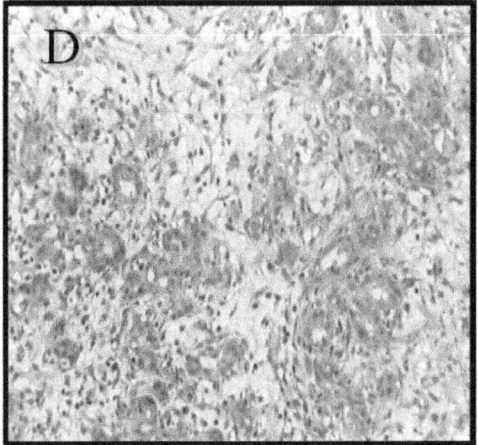

C: 12 hours after 3 % sodium taurocholate injection into PBD with the histo-pathological changes: Interstitial edema, inflammatory infiltration and acinar cell necrosis (sublobular and lobular) (H.E. x 100)

D: 72 hours after 3 % sodium taurocholate injection into PBD with the histo-pathological changes: Severe loss of acinar cells, intense inflammatory infiltration and fibrosis (H.E. x 100)

Light microscopic pictures of the pancreas from the taurocholate dose response study

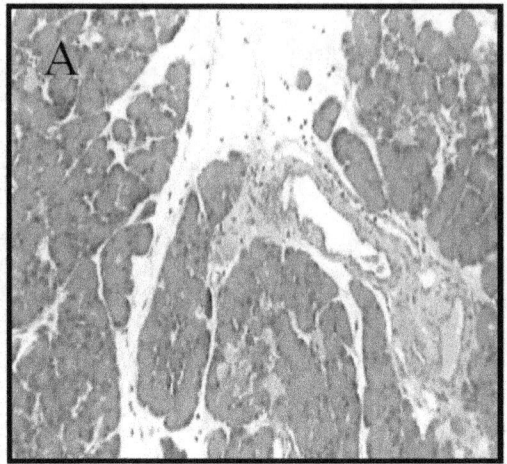

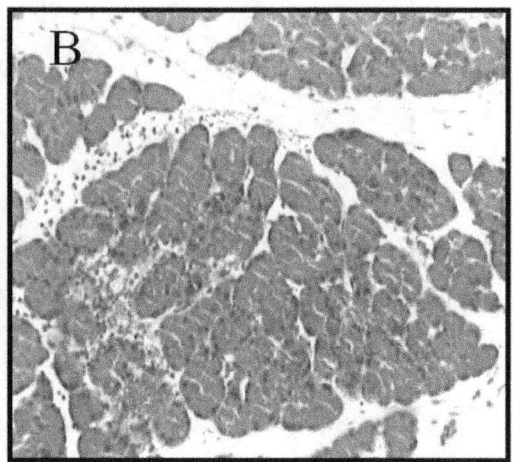

A: 6 hours after isotonic saline injection into PBD with the histo-pathological changes: Interstitial edema, slight inflammatory infiltration but no acinar cell necrosis (H.E. x 100)

B: 6 hours after 1 % sodium taurocholate injection into PBD with the histo-pathological changes: Interstitial edema, slight inflammatory infiltration but no acinar cell necrosis (H.E. x 100)

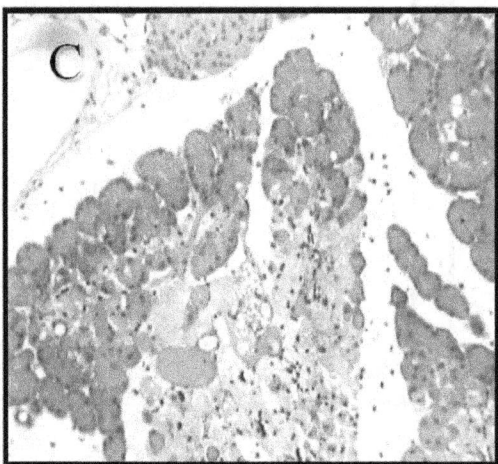

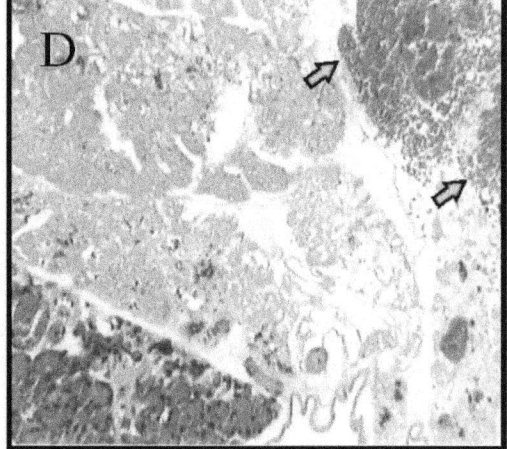

C: 6 hours after 3 % sodium taurocholate injection into PBD with the histo-pathological changes: Interstitial edema, inflammatory infiltration and sublobular necrosis (H.E. x 100)

D: 6 hours after 6 % sodium taurocholate injection into PBD with the histo-pathological changes: Interstitial edema, inflammatory infiltration, severe lobular necrosis and severe haemorrhages (arrows) (H.E. x 100)

Light microscopic pictures of the pancreas from the cerulein time course study

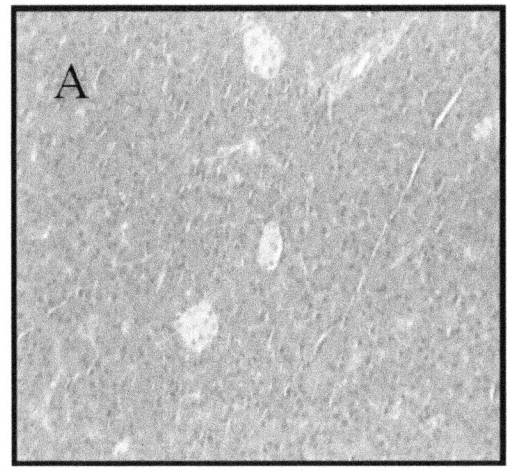

A: Normal pancreas from control animals (H.E. x 100)

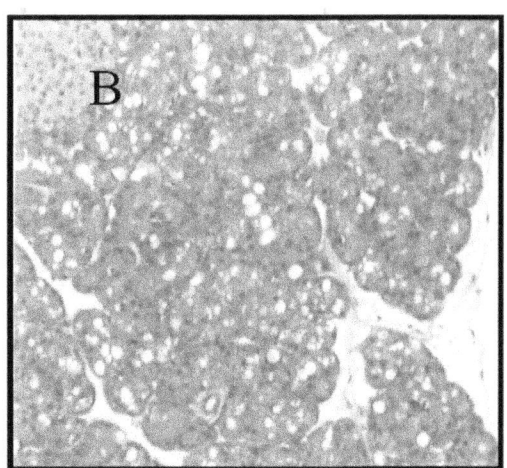

B: 3 hours of cerulein infusion (10 µg/kg/h) with the hisopathological changes: interstitial edema and some vacoulization in the acini (H.E. x 100).

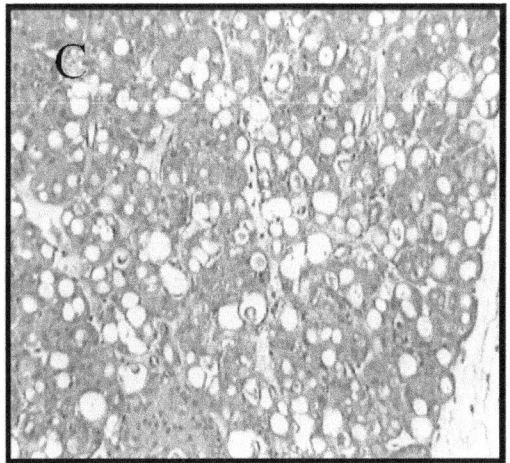

C: 12 hours of cerulein infusion (10 µg/kg/h) and the histopathological changes: Interstitial edema, inflammatory infiltration and remarkable acinar vacuolization (H.E. x 100)

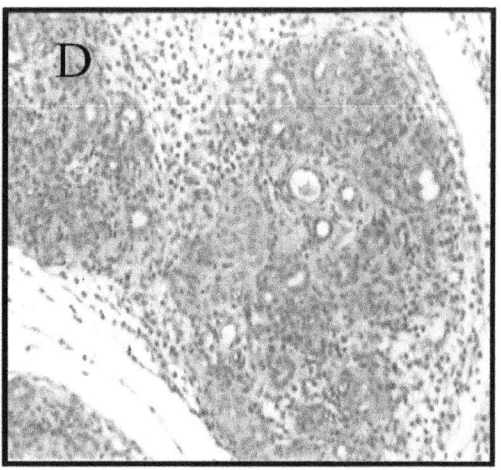

D: 72 hours of cerulein infusion (10 µg/kg/h) and the histopathological changes: Severe inflammatory infiltration, loss of acinar cells and still some interstitial edema (H.E. x 100)